DEVELOPMENTAL DYSPHASIA

Developmental Dysphasia

Edited by

MARIA A. WYKE

Department of Psychology
The National Hospitals for Nervous Diseases
Maida Vale, London W9 ITL

1978

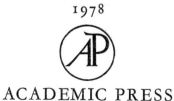

ACADEMIC PRESS
London · New York · San Francisco

A Subsidiary of Harcourt Brace Jovanovich, Publishers

ACADEMIC PRESS INC. (LONDON) LTD.
24/28 Oval Road
London NW1

United States Edition published by
ACADEMIC PRESS INC.
111 Fifth Avenue
New York, New York 10003

Library of Congress Catalog Card Number: 78-52102
ISBN: 0-12-766950-7

PRINTED IN GREAT BRITAIN BY
LATIMER TREND & COMPANY LTD PLYMOUTH

LIST OF CONTRIBUTORS

Arthur L. Benton Department of Neurology, University of Iowa Hospital and Clinics, Iowa City, Iowa 52242, U.S.A.

Jean M. Cooper National Hospitals College of Speech Sciences, 59 Portland Place, London W1N 3AJ, England

Richard F. Cromer M.R.C. Developmental Psychology Unit, Drayton House, Gordon Street, London WC1H 0AN, England

Pauline Griffiths National Hospitals College of Speech Sciences, 59 Portland Place, London W1N 3AJ, England

Paula Menyuk School of Education, Boston University, 765 Commonwealth Avenue, Boston, Mass. 02215, U.S.A.

Malcolm Piercy Psychological Laboratory, University of Cambridge, Cambridge, England

Isabelle Rapin Neurology and Pedriatrics (Neurology), The Saul R. Korey Department of Neurology, Albert Einstein College of Medicine of Yeshiva University, 1300 Morris Park Avenue, Bronx, N.Y. 10461, U.S.A.

Paula Tallal Instructor in Pedriatrics, John F. Kennedy Institute, 707 North Broadway, Baltimore, Maryland 21205, U.S.A.

Barbara C. Wilson Department of Neurology, North Shore University Hospital – Cornell University Medical College, Manhasset, N.Y. 11030, U.S.A.

Oliver L. Zangwill Psychological Labaratory, University of Cambridge, Cambridge, England

PREFACE

Developmental dysphasia, i.e. the deficit in the acquisition of normal language functions in children of normal or above normal intelligence and with adequate hearing ability to permit the perception of verbal sounds, has attracted considerable attention for a number of years. The problem has engaged the interest of scientists from very different fields, and many attempts have been made to unravel the essential nature of the disability. For a long time the deficits of children with developmental dysphasia had been merely observed and recorded, but lately there has been an increased number of investigations which have viewed developmental dysphasia in the light of more rigorous experimental procedures.

This book contains chapters devoted to the discussion of our current understanding of developmental dysphasia. The approach is multi-disciplinary and the volume assembles contributions from neurologists, psychologists, linguists, speech therapists and remedial teachers, all of whom have had close contact with this problem.

The first chapter is intended as an introduction dealing with the concept of developmental dysphasia, attempting to delineate the boundaries of this complex disorder. In the remaining chapters the authors provide up-to-date accounts and critical evaluation of work which has been carried out in their respective fields. They also present their own researches and discuss the theoretical implications of their findings.

The question of the essential nature of developmental dysphasis is far from being answered, but it is hoped that the pages of this book may point the way to many future research developments in this area.

The Editor would like to thank Miss A. Greenwood, Mr Piers Ashworth and Dr G. Schott for their invaluable assistance.

May 1978   MARIA A. WYKE

CONTENTS

The Concept of
Developmental Dysphasia

O. L. Zangwill

The term *developmental dysphasia* has come into general use to denote slow, limited or otherwise faulty development of language in children who do not otherwise give evidence of gross neurological or psychiatric disability. Accordingly, children with infantile hemiplegia or other forms of cerebral palsy are not normally classed as cases of developmental aphasia, even though their speech may be slow to develop and present various types of abnormality. Much the same is true of mentally handicapped or autistic children. In general, lack or impairment of speech secondary to deafness is likewise excluded from the category of developmental dysphasia, though it should be borne in mind that some degree of auditory defect, in particular high frequency deafness, may be found in some children who have been diagnosed as aphasic. On the whole, however, it may be said that the outstanding handicap of developmental dysphasia is social and educational rather than physical, and that sensory or motor defects of any severity are seldom in evidence.

The Syndrome of Developmental Dysphasia

What, then, is developmental dysphasia? According to Ingram (1976), it is a condition in which, in spite of normal intelligence and unexceptional home background, the child is slow to develop speech and such speech as he has acquired is marked by defective articulation of certain groups of speech sounds, in particular consonant sounds. Speech output is commonly limited both in amount and syntactical structure and sense of rhythm is typically poor. While the nature of the disorder varies a good deal from one child to another, Ingram has pointed out that its general pattern is on the whole consistent and follows that of normal speech development; it is the speech sounds that are acquired relatively late that are most prone to omission or substitution. Oral comprehension is as a rule normal, except in very severe cases or in those in which hearing loss is appreciable. Even where comprehension appears unaffected, however, sophisticated methods of examination may disclose subtle impairment. As is well known, developmental language disorders are much more common in boys than in girls, and according to Ingram, the ratio varies in different series of patients from between 2-to-1 and 5-to-1 in favour of the male. This, together with the not infrequent incidence of similar disorders in other members of the same family, has commonly been taken to indicate that genetic factors play a very real part in the origins of this condition.

As dysphasic children grow older, educational handicaps soon become apparent. These are most prominent in connection with learning to read and spell and, unless their speech handicap is obviously still severe, such children are often classified as 'dyslexic' – as though difficulty in learning to read and spell is something quite different from that of learning to speak. If a reliable history can be obtained, dyslexic children are usually found to have been relatively late in starting to talk and minor difficulties in articulation or speech output can often be shown to exist (Miles, 1974). Further, intelligence as assessed by 'verbal' test batteries is commonly, though not invariably, significantly below that as assessed by 'non-verbal' test batteries, which lay stress on visual and manipulative skills (Kinsbourne and Warrington, 1963). Less widely appreciated, perhaps, are the striking difficulties which dyslexic children so commonly experience in verbal learning, especially in rote learning. This is shown particularly well in learning to spell, but it is often equally apparent in learning poetry or indeed the multiplication tables. Fortunately, semantic memory is largely if not completely spared.

When the child proceeds to secondary school, it is not surprising that he typically finds English, French and Latin are the subjects which give him the greatest trouble and here even quite minor dysphasic difficulties come to assume major importance. Fortunately, comprehension and semantic memory are usually good enough to make possible acceptable progress in subjects such as history and geography, as sometimes also in science, particularly in biology. Interestingly enough, mathematics is seldom affected and some dyslexic children become talented mathematicians. None the less, many highly intelligent and industrious school-children with dyslexic and kindred troubles come hopelessly to grief over written examinations and few succeed in gaining admission to university or can confidently look forward to a professional career.

In spite of speech therapy and the kindred forms of remedial education now available, many children suffering from developmental dysphasia remain handicapped as adults. As might be expected, occupational placement is often a matter of the utmost difficulty. No matter how intelligent, few children with appreciable dysphasia or even merely dyslexic difficulties are able to find employment commensurate with their intelligence, and all too little attention has hitherto been given to the problems of employment of the dysphasic adult.

Three Illustrative Cases

Three cases may be briefly described. The first is one of the earliest ever to be reported at any length in this country. It was communicated by Sir Henry Head (1926) as an example of semantic aphasia of congenital origin and illustrates well the problems of an intelligent adult handicapped since childhood by a developmental language disorder.

Case 1 (Head (1926) Case no. 25)
The patient, aged 43 when first seen by Head, was a professional horticulturist and a woman of evident intelligence and culture. She had been educated privately and her father, a school inspector, was well aware of her disabilities and had taken endless trouble over her education. Even so, she was thirteen before she had learned to read. After she grew up, she worked for a time in educational administration but was obliged to abandon it owing to her difficulty in writing and expressing her thoughts in a coherent manner. She was definitely right-handed and no history of birth complications or of kindred language difficulties in other members of the family is recorded. There were no abnormal signs on general or neurological examination. Head reports that this patient's articulate speech was adequate in conversation and that she had no difficulty in finding words or names. When tired or under stress, however, she developed a marked stammer. Understanding of speech was on the whole intact though some errors were made in carrying out commands, in particular those involving discrimination of right and left. The patient complained however, that she was often unable to hold in her mind a task explained to her in the course of conversation, which clearly suggests a degree of impairment in short-term verbal memory. Although she could read well aloud, she was liable to miss the general significance of a story if she read it silently.

According to Head, this lady's 'congenital defect in symbolic expression' was more marked and disabling in written expression. Whereas she would write adequately at a simple level, any attempt to express general ideas is said to have led to profound deterioration. Her spelling, always poor, suffered in much the same way; the harder the task the worse it became until the faults 'reached a degree unknown in an educated person'. Thus in describing her difficulties on a test of writing single words to dictation, she wrote 'cissors and penny difficult because one must choose between alternatives and there is knothing to guid'. A propos of her mis-spelling of "nothing", she wrote: 'This is excellent for showy (showing) up what goes on'. In writing down what she remembered of a short passage her version read: 'The writer is in italy and tels of his garden in which he has fig trees, vines, pomgranates and many other things'. She could do simple arithmetic using pencil and paper without difficulty but her mental arithmetic was slow and un-certain and she even had difficulty in appreciating the relative value of coins.

Apart from these essentially linguistic disabilities, this lady also appeared to have suffered from a certain weakness in copying, drawing and topographical orientation. She had difficulty in following directions as to routes and her drawings of ground-plans were decidedly poor. She also made errors in telling the time and in setting the hands of a clock to the time specified by the examiner. Further, she confessed to great difficulty in understanding pictorial jokes, with or without captions.

This is a relatively mild case of developmental dysphasia in an in-telligent adult in whom the principal difficulties were mainly, though not exclusively, confined to writing and spelling. Today, it might be classified as developmental dyslexia rather than dysphasia, and a rather similar case has been described under this title by the present writer (Zangwill, 1960). This was a girl of 15 who in addition to severe backwardness in reading and spelling had striking deficiencies in drawing, copying and spatial orientation. Like Head's patient, she had difficulty in regard to left and right and in telling the time. Although right-handed, there was some left-handedness in her family. Cases of this kind show clearly that the symbolic disorder may interpenetrate the spatial environment thus giving rise to quite extensive intellectual handicap.

The next two cases are personal ones and have been chosen to illustrate two important points. First, the familial incidence of developmental language disorders and, secondly, the links between slow speech develop-ment in childhood and difficulties in reading and writing later on: possible links between ambilaterality and dyslexia are also indicated. The first case is that of a predominantly left-handed boy with marked reading and spelling backwardness who had been relatively slow in learning to talk and still had a trace of difficulty in articulation. His father and grandfather had had similar though possibly less severe educational difficulties. There was no reason to suggest minimal brain damage at birth or in early childhood.

Case 2

This 11-year-old boy was referred by his grandmother, a retired medical practitioner, who had become concerned about his educational prospects. She related that both her husband who had been in the Church, and her son, had been very poor readers and spellers and she was worried lest the condition were hereditary and liable to become worse in successive generations. This boy was brought to see me by his father who was manager of a small retail business. The father stated that he had himself been much handicapped at school by his very poor reading and spelling and had failed to pass any examinations. His son's birth had been entirely normal but he had been relatively slow in learning to walk and to talk, and his attempts at learning to read were at first so deplorable that his mother had thought that he must be educationally subnormal, a view shared by his then headmaster and by an educational psychologist. He was having considerable difficulties at school.

On examination, the boy proved to be predominantly left-handed though there was otherwise no left-handedness on either side of the family. Manipulation was clumsy and there was a trace of difficulty in articulation. The WISC IQ was 117, the verbal IQ being 14 points below the performance IQ There was a discrepancy of three and a half years between chronological age and attainment level on the Schonell reading and spelling tests. It was ascertained that the father's IQ fell within one point of his son's, but his scores on the Schonell attainment tests were at an average level.

The third case is that of a right-handed though partly ambilateral boy with a severe dyslexic handicap. Both his father and a paternal uncle had been poor readers and spellers, and there was likewise some indication of reading and spelling trouble on his mother's side of the family, though she herself was unaffected. Two of his three brothers had difficulties similar to, though somewhat less severe, than his own. I was alerted to the case by the boy's mother, the wife of a physician, who wrote me an unsolicited letter in which she said 'You might conceivably be short of research material in the form of dyslexic children; if so, I feel our family could provide you with a rich hunting-ground'.

Case 3
A very full history of this boy, then 15 years old, was provided by his parents. They reported that birth and delivery had been entirely normal and there were no complications of any kind. He had been a little slow in learning to talk and his speech was 'cluttered'; later on, he developed a mild hesitant stammer. Although right-handed, as an infant he had shown some left-hand tendencies, to an extent which had led his father to believe that he would eventually become left-handed. However, he is now somewhat ambilateral although predominantly dextral.

In learning to read, this boy was reported to have made many reversals, particularly with numerals. His early progress at school was so unsatisfactory that, like Case 2, he was at first suspected of being educationally subnormal. Fortunately, a child psychiatrist who saw him at the age of 8 considered that he had a specific disability in the visuo-motor sphere. At this age his WISC IQ was 115, with a reading age of 5·6 and an arithmetic age of 6·6. His drawing was said to be of very poor quality and he obtained a mental age equivalent of only 6 years on the Goodenough tests.

This boy had been fortunate in having been educated mainly at private schools at which remedial help had been available. By age 10 reading age had risen to 7·3 years and arithmetic age to 7·5 years. He has since continued to make progress and has recently proceeded to a public school which makes some provision for backward readers. His remedial English teacher reports that he still reverses some letters in writing and shortens words. But none the less he has made quite a promising start.

Regarding familial incidence, the following points are of interest.

1. His father stated that as a boy he had had relatively severe writing and spelling problems which had not, however, prevented him from qualifying in medicine though he had had great difficulty in passing his examinations. His verbal learning had always been poor and written composition slow and effortful. Indeed as a medical student he had worked out a special technique to enable him to write examination answers as quickly and concisely as possible. He reported some diffi-culty in visualising words and was apt easily to lose the place in reading, often tracking with his forefinger. Apart from poor spelling and rela-tively uncertain auditory memory, he had managed to cope effectively with his work as a rural general practitioner.

2. One of the boy's paternal uncles was reported to be ambilateral and a poor speller who had had difficulties similar to those of his brother at school, more especially with language subjects.

3. The boy's mother had at no time difficulty with reading or spelling but informed us that both her father and one of her brothers were stammerers. This and one other brother had also had difficulty with reading and spelling.

4. Two of the boy's younger brothers were likewise dyslexic although less markedly so than himself. His youngest brother is still too young for one to be able to assess his reading capacity.

This family resembles several of those reported by S. T. Orton (1937), who is rightly regarded as a pioneer of paediatric neurology. Although the speech disorders were relatively unimportant, the severe difficulties with reading and spelling had most serious educational implications, and were quite possibly also of occupational significance in adult life.

Of particular interest to the lay reader is Elizabeth Browning's account of the case of her own son (Browning, 1972), who developed a severe developmental dysphasia with partial deafness as the outcome of early brain injury. Her account illustrates well the difficulties encountered by many parents in connection with the diagnosis and remedial treatment of dysphasic difficulties in children as well as the problems that arise later on in regard to education and occupational placement.

Auditory Defect in Aphasia

In 1930, A W. G. Ewing produced a short monograph on aphasia in children to which Dr (later Lord) Adrian contributed an appreciative introduction. Its purpose was to direct attention to the selective incidence of high frequency deafness in a small group of children diagnosed as cases either of aphasia or of 'congenital auditory imperception', by which name receptive language disorders were at that time widely known. Of the 10 patients tested, the audiometric findings fell within the distribution for normal control children in four cases whereas in the remaining six there was an apparently severe defect of hearing limited only to sounds of high frequency. In the latter cases, only the readings from the responses in the lower frequencies tested (256 v.d. and below) fell within the distribution for the children of normal hearing. In consequence, Ewing was led to conclude that the apparent aphasia in the cases with high frequency deafness is in no sense a true disorder of speech or language but purely a form of retardation consequent upon selectively impaired hearing capacity.

What of the four children who showed no apparent abnormality of hearing? Here, too, Ewing was dissatisfied with the diagnosis of 'aphasia' though for a rather different reason. He maintained that there was no convincing parallel between their language difficulties and those of adults who had acquired their aphasia through damage to the brain. Not only is the degree of variability in the clinical picture much greater in the latter than in the former but the mistakes in speech made by these children are typical of those made by normal children at certain stages of development. He therefore concluded that there are fundamental distinctions both in symptoms and aetiology between failures of natural speech development in childhood and the breakdown of the perfected processes of language and communication in later life.

Ewing may be regarded as the originator of the concept of 'cerebral immaturity' or 'developmental lag' in relation to childhood language disorder. This concept is widely accepted today and Ewing deserves great credit for detaching developmental speech disorder from what Critchley (1970) has termed the 'aphasiological context' and relating it to retardation

in language development and language learning generally. At the same
time, the role of hearing loss in developmental dysphasia obviously calls
for reassessment in the light of more recent work. In a series of children
aged between 3 and 6 referred to hospital for very slow speech development, Ingram (1976) reports that almost 10 per cent had serious hearing
loss. He also warns that even with sophisticated apparatus and much experience, a definitive diagnosis of hearing loss is often difficult. This
matter is discussed by Isabelle Rapin and Barbara Wilson in the following
chapter. In particular, the authors stress the readiness with which high
frequency deafness can be overlooked and the need for repeated testing
before a firm diagnosis can be confidently made. They also direct attention
to the very varying degree to which hearing loss affects language development in different children. Whereas some are severely affected by only
moderate degrees of hearing loss others, albeit with more severe degrees
of deafness, none the less develop adequate speech despite their defective
articulation. Finally, they make the very valid point that conditions which
cause acquired hearing loss in newborn babies may also cause primary
damage to the brain mechanisms underlying the acquisition and control
of speech.

Since Ewing's day, a number of methods of detecting hearing loss other
than those of classical audiometry have been devised. Later in this book
Richard Cromer considers in some detail the work of Mark and Hardy
(1958) on disturbances of the orienting response to sound in language
handicapped children and some of the difficulties that arise in its interpretation. Following Eisenson (1968), he suggests that dysphasic children may
have a defect not in the perception of sound *per se* but in the perception of
sounds in appropriate phonetic contexts. That some more subtle defect
may exist at the acoustic feature analysis stage of perception is likewise
suggested by Paula Tallal and Malcolm Piercy in their chapter on defects
of auditory perception in children with developmental dysphasia. On the
basis of some of their own experimental work, they direct special attention
to the difficulty experienced by many such children in processing rapidly
changing acoustic information. This may well prove a primary disability
in language impaired children and is deserving of closer study.

Sequential Order in Speech

In 1951, Karl Lashley published a seminal paper on the problem of serial
order in behaviour. While treating it as a basic issue in neurobiology
generally, he placed special emphasis on speech as a prime example of
temporal integration and psychologists have not been slow to build upon
his example. It is, moreover, a problem that has attracted particular

interest in its bearings on disorders of language. While defects in the appreciation or learning of serial order have been reported by many investigators (see e.g. Doehring, 1968), it has been comparatively little discussed in relation to developmental aphasia. In this volume, however, it has come to occupy an important place.

In his chapter on the cognitive abilities of children with developmental aphasia (p. 43), Arthur Benton addresses himself to the problem of whether the defects of sequencing which have been so often described in language disordered children are of a general nature or whether, on the other hand, they are specific to the auditory modality. Although the evidence is somewhat conflicting, he considers that the defect, if not wholly restricted to audition, is at any rate most prominent in this modality. In common with Paula Tallal and Malcolm Piercy (p. 63), he believes that it constitutes a 'distinctive defect in the auditory perception of children with receptive-expressive dysphasia'. On the other hand, Richard Cromer (p. 85) is less confident of this degree of specificity. He thinks less in terms of a defect in the auditory modality than of an impairment within the linguistic system itself. That is to say, developmental dysphasia is a defect not of sensory reception nor yet of higher level auditory processing but of language proper.

The hypothesis advanced by Cromer is based upon the analysis of the written language abilities of a group of dysphasic children as compared with those of a comparable group of deaf children. As he points out, the two groups differed appreciably in the nature of the difficulties they respectively encountered. Whereas the deaf children tried a variety of syntactical structures, including some which relied on complex transformations, the dysphasic children are thought to have failed to use the kind of structures that would involve a true hierarchical organisation of the whole sentence. In short, they suffer from a hierarchical ordering deficit.

It is evident that these three chapters indicate that there are important differences in approach between the psychological and linguistic points of view. Whereas the psychologist seeks to base his models upon relatively circumscribed experimental findings, the linguist is more concerned to establish a general theory of language disorder. Each has much to learn from the other's approach.

Cerebral Dominance in Dysphasia

Over the past fifty years, many authors have directed attention to the prevalence of left-handedness or lack of strong and/or consistent lateral preferences among children with speech disorders or backwardness in reading (Zangwill, 1962). Some have also commented upon the frequency of left-handedness in the families of such children, even if they themselves appear to be fully right-handed (Naidoo, 1972; Ingram, 1976). In general, weak, mixed or inconsistent lateral preferences are the most frequent finding: Ingram and Reid (1956) for instance directed attention to this feature in 71 per cent of a large group of patients diagnosed as cases of developmental aphasia, and Harris (1957) reported a significantly higher proportion of mixed-hand preferences in a group of dyslexic children as compared with a randomly selected control group.

The tendency to left-handedness or mixed handedness both in children with developmental speech, reading and writing disorders and/or in their families led Orton (1937) to postulate that developmental language disability is caused by a lack of clear-cut cerebral dominance, i.e. a failure to lateralise language exclusively to one or other hemisphere. This he believed to result in the frequency of reversal of letters or syllables in reading and writing, more rarely in mirror writing or the transposition of syllables in oral speech ('backward speech'). While the theory put forward by Orton to explain these phenomena has seldom been taken very seriously, he none the less deserves great credit for being the first to link backwardness in speech and reading with factors in the ontogeny of cerebral dominance.

Although not all who are interested in developmental dysphasia attach comparable importance to the laterality factor (e.g. Sparrow and Satz, 1970), it is none the less plausible to assume that the 'developmental lag' which in the absence of gross brain damage is generally held to underlie developmental aphasia, has its neural correlate in slow, faulty or incomplete lateralisation of language processes. Even Sparrow and Satz (1970), while failing to find significant differences between dyslexic and control groups in respect of hand preference and manual dexterity, as for that matter in familial history of left-handedness, do in fact find that their dyslexic children had a higher frequency of left-ear advantage on a dichotic listening task. This led them to postulate greater participation in speech on the part of the right cerebral hemisphere in the backward than in the normal reader. It is also of some interest that Hécaen and Sauget (1971) postulate a higher degree of 'cerebral ambilaterality' in cases of acquired aphasia in left-handers in which there is a high incidence of familial sinistrality.

In the light of these considerations, it appears likely that issues of cerebral dominance will come to throw light on the neurology of developmental aphasia as they have in the past on that of acquired aphasia. This would appear an obvious target for future research.

References

Browning, E. (1972). 'I Can't See What You're Saying'. Elek, London.

Critchley, M. (1970). 'The Dyslexic Child'. Heinemann, London.

Doehring, D. G. (1968). 'Patterns of Impairment in Specific Reading Disability'. Indiana University Press.

Eisenson, J. (1968). Developmental aphasia: A speculative view with therapeutic implications. *J. Speech Hear. Dis.* **33**, 3–13.

Ewing, A. W. G. (1930). 'Aphasia in Childhood'. Oxford University Press, London.

Harris, A. J. (1957). Lateral dominance, directional confusion and reading disability. *J. Psychol.* **44**, 283–294.

Head, H. (1926). 'Aphasia and Kindred Disorders of Speech', Vol. 2. Cambridge University Press, London.

Hécaen, H. and Sauget, J. (1971). Cerebral dominance in left-handed subjects. *Cortex* **7**, 19–48.

Ingram, T. T. S. (1976). Speech Disorders in Childhood. *In* 'Foundations of Language Development' (E. H. and Elizabeth Lenneberg, eds), Vol. 2, pp. 295–261. Academic Press, New York. Unesco, Paris.

Ingram, T. T. S. and Reid, J. F. (1956). Developmental aphasia observed in a department of child psychiatry. *Arch. Dis. Childh.* **31**, 162–172.

Kinsbourne, M. and Warrington, E. K. (1963). Developmental factors in reading and writing backwardness. *Brit. J. Psychol.* **54**, 145–156.

Lashley, K. S. (1951). The problem of serial order in behavior. *In* 'Cerebral Mechanisms in Behavior' (L. A. Jeffress, ed.), pp. 112–136. Wiley, New York.

Mark, H. J. and Hardy, W. G. (1958). Orienting reflex disturbances in central auditory or language handicapped children. *J. Speech Hear. Dis.* **23**, 237–242.

Miles, T. R. (1974). 'The Dyslexic Child'. Priory Press, London.

Naidoo, S. (1972). 'Specific Dyslexia'. Pitman, London.

Orton, S. T. (1937). 'Reading, Writing and Speech Problems in Children'. Chapman and Hall, London.

Sparrow, S. and Satz, P. (1970). Dyslexia, laterality and neuropsychological development. *In* 'Specific Reading Disability: Advances in Theory and Method' (D. J. Bakker and P. Satz, eds). Rotterdam University Press.

Zangwill, O. L. (1960). 'Cerebral Dominance and its Relation to Psychological Function'. Oliver and Boyd, Edinburgh.

Zangwill, O. L. (1962). Dyslexia in relation to cerebral dominance. *In* 'Reading Disability: Progress and Research Needs in Dyslexia' (J. Money, ed.), pp. 103–114. The Johns Hopkins Press, Baltimore.

Children with Developmental Language Disability: Neurological Aspects and Assessment

Isabelle Rapin and Barbara C. Wilson

Disorders of language function result from deficits at the level of receiving, processing, and/or expressing language, and our basic assumption throughout this chapter is that failure to develop language is always, except in rare instances of extreme environmental deprivation, the consequence of neurological dysfunction affecting pathways which transmit information from the ear to the brain, within the brain itself, or from the brain to the muscles of articulation.

Language is composed of a series of arbitrary symbols. It is a vehicle for thinking and for the communication of thought (Piaget, 1963; Morehead and Morehead, 1974). Language is socially derived and transmissible and it conforms to a fixed set of rules. The relationship between these linguistic rules (grammar) and neurophysiological function is still a subject of debate. We shall here define a child as having a developmental language disability if he fails to develop and use language for communication, providing that hearing loss, cognitive and motor deficits and behavioural disorders are judged insufficient to account for the extent of the language impairment.

The aural-oral channel is not the only possible language pathway. We know that language can be transmitted to the brain through visual and somatosensory channels, and be expressed both manually and orally. Some children, particularly those with a defective acoustic channel, will develop, to some extent, alternative channels for communication, usually a visual-manual one, whilst other children seem totally unable to process symbols through any channel. This latter group suffers from the most severe of language disabilities, and since they have essentially no means for communication they often appear withdrawn, i.e. 'autistic'. Fortunately, most children with developmental language disability exhibit a less profound impairment of symbolic communication.

13

We hold the view, which is shared by others (Ingram, 1959; Morley, 1972; Rees, 1973; Aram and Nation, 1975; Kerschensteiner and Huber, 1975), that there are multiple syndromes of developmental language disability. It is unlikely that a single deficit would account for the many aspects of developmental language disorders encountered in the clinic. Furthermore, it appears that some children who are delayed in acquiring language may not be suffering from a lesion in the central nervous system, but rather from a delay in the maturation of relevant neurological systems. Rather than exhibiting deviant patterns of language development, these children's language may follow a normal developmental sequence, but at a significantly slower pace (Menyuk, 1974). The present state of knowledge does not always enable us to differentiate between possible aetiologies or to give a definite prognosis as to the outcome of such disabilities, at least in early childhood.

Not all children whose language acquisition is delayed or deviant can be considered to have a primary language disability. We cannot stress too strongly that the two most common reasons for children's failure to learn to speak are peripheral hearing loss and mental retardation. While it is possible that severe emotional disability related to an unfavourable environmental situation might retard the acquisition of language, we have found that behavioural disorders exhibited by non-speaking children are more likely to be the consequence rather than the cause of their inadequate communication.

The Role of the Paediatric Neurologist

Among the professionals who will evaluate a child who fails to develop language, the responsibility for the medical aspects of the problem rests primarily with the paediatric neurologist. The neurologist's background and training enable him to assess the clinical history, particularly the events surrounding pregnancy, birth, and the neonatal period, which may have played a role in pathogenesis. The neurologist's knowledge of genetics is an aid in the interpretation of data from the family background. His examination of the child will focus on the assessment of the development of motor, social, adaptive and cognitive skills, as well as the child's communicative ability. As he evaluates the child, two separate themes will be foremost in his mind: localisation and pathogenesis.

First we will consider where in the communication channel, from the ear, to the brain, to the mechanisms of oral speech, things may have gone wrong. What components of this system, required for the processing of aural-oral messages, may be malfunctioning? This first question is essentially a systems question, seeking to define in neuropsychological terms those operations which may be defective and those anatomo-physiological dysfunctions which may be responsible for the defective operation. The second question is one of pathogenesis: what may have caused this break-down? What kind of brain insult has the child sustained? Is the problem static, or progressive? Is it possible that minor seizures, caused by a primary lesion, might interfere with cortical functioning and that language could improve if the seizures were controlled? Is the cause more likely to be a developmental delay, a malformation, or an acquired lesion? Could the problem be genetic? The neurologist will also ask himself whether environmental factors may have played a significant role. Are the child's needs for warmth and emotional support adequately met? Does his environment supply stimulating material for his exploring mind? Is he being spoken to? Is there more than one language used in the home?

In some ways, one can look upon the investigation carried out by the child neurologist as a primary screening. The role of this physician who usually sees the child only once or perhaps twice, is to sample from a wide range of behaviours and to consider all possible causes of pathogenetic mechanisms. This will assist other professionals to centre their explorations on areas which appear most likely to yield relevant information to explain the child's failure to acquire language, and to define an appropriate educational approach

Before discussing the examination techniques available to the child neurologist, it is important first to consider the aural-oral communication system and the types of disorders which are likely to interfere with its function, since the system and its disorders constitute the framework for the neurologist's investigation.

The Auditory-Verbal Communication System

The analysis of the disorders of this system in children will be dealt with under the following headings:
1 Disorders of input through the acoustic channel:
  (a) Hearing impairment.
  (b) Disorders of auditory perception (e.g. duration, pattern, order, etc.)
  (c) Disorders affecting the decoding of the phonological aspects of speech (verbal auditory agnosia).
2 Disorders of linguistic processing:
  (a) Disorders of language and hemispheric specialisation (hemispheric asymmetry).
  (b) Syndromes in children with deficient language development.
  (c) Disorders of language: the role of short-term auditory memory.

3 General disorders of brain function which may affect language acquisition:
  (*a*) Hyperkinetic syndrome.
  (*b*) Autism.
  (*c*) Deficits in cognitive competence.
4 Disorders of speech output:
  (*a*) Defective syntactic programming.
  (*b*) Defective phonemic programming.
  (*c*) Dysarthria.
  (*d*) Stuttering.

The above outline is not to be interpreted as suggesting that a single specific deficit is likely to be the cause of the linguistic dysfunction, or that this deficit will be isolated and that no other evidence of brain dysfunction will be found. On the contrary, our experience is that 'pure' syndromes are in fact exceptional: we often find evidence of dysfunction for behaviours which do not appear directly relevant to linguistic acquisition (for instance, delays of gross motor development such as walking, visuo-motor problems, poor visual memory, difficulty with non-verbal analogical reasoning, etc.). While these deficits are useful confirmatory evidence for cerebral dysfunction and may lead the neurologist and neuropsychologist to hypotheses regarding localisation of brain dysfunction, they are unlikely to be directly relevant to the pathogenesis of the linguistic deficit. They reflect the extent of the cerebral dysfunction but are irrelevant to the language disorder itself.

Disorders of Acoustic Input

HEARING IMPAIRMENT

In the authors' clinical experience, the single most common error in investigating a child who fails to develop language is to overlook a peripheral hearing loss. This statement may come as a surprise to those who are not aware of the enormous difficulties encountered in assessing hearing in a very young, handicapped and uncooperative child.

There are two basic approaches to testing hearing – behavioural tests and physiological tests. The first approach, which is also the most useful, precise and widely used, tests the child's ability to emit a specific gesture indicating that he has heard a certain sound. The advantage of this method is that it tests the entire acoustic pathway, from the peripheral receptor, through the peripheral and central auditory pathway, to the processing of the acoustic message and its use in programming a specific output. It is a test of the whole system as it is presumably used in everyday life.

There are problems in using behavioural audiometric techniques with young children, especially with a non-speaking child. One has to be sure that the child understands what is wanted, that he will produce with reliability the prescribed gesture, and that he is able to focus his attention and remain motivated to respond. That is to say the child is being asked to participate in a psychophysical procedure. One can use conditioning techniques to train most pre-school children to respond to a specific stimulus and, with appropriate reinforcement, one can keep motivation and attention levels high. Play audiometry (Barr, 1955), the peep show (Dix and Hallpike, 1947) and reaction time (Rapin and Steinherz, 1970) are examples of such approaches to behavioural audiometry. In the very young child, and when handicaps make conditioned behavioural approaches inapplicable, one is forced to resort to non-conditioned behavioural responses. These may include startle reactions to loud sound, orienting responses towards the sound source, and changes in facial expression or levels of activity. In infants, other methods are also used, such as awakening from sleep (Wedenberg, 1956), changes in activity (Simmons and Russ, 1974) or heart rate (Steinschneider et al., 1966). These methods are laborious, and multiple tests are required in order to ascertain that results are reliable. Even when results are considered reliable they may reflect threshold of response but not threshold of hearing (auditory sensitivity).

When behavioural audiometry is impossible or unreliable, one must turn to physiological measures of hearing. The most widely used are the recording of the stapedius reflex in response to loud sound, cochleography, and EEG auditory evoked response audiometry. They do not require cooperation on the part of the child and are therefore applicable to infants and to the multiple handicapped and uncooperative child. They give no information, however, on the ability to process sound and use it to programme behaviour. Results of physiological tests must be confirmed by behavioural audiometry and long-term assessments.

Measurements of impedance make it possible to study the mechanical characteristics of the middle ear (Wilber, 1974), and are very useful indicators for Eustachian tube dysfunction associated with fluid in the middle ear – a very common condition in children. Fluid in the middle ear has a significant effect upon audition, especially if the child is already hard of hearing; one may speculate in addition that it is harmful to children with an acoustic processing disorder. When acoustic impedance is normal or reasonably normal and there is no facial paralysis, the lack of reflex contraction of the stapedius muscle in response to sound is an indication that hearing is impaired. Although this test does not provide threshold values, it does give independent evidence of hearing function. Cochleography (Crowley et al., 1975), is the recording of electrophysiological responses of the hair cells, acoustic nerve, and brain stem relay nuclei to sound (Picton *et al.*, 1974). Special equipment is required to record these responses. The child must be sedated, but the data seem to provide information as to the site of the dysfunction. EEG-evoked response audiometry may depend on the recording of early responses (Mendel, 1974), presumably originating in the auditory cortex, or later, more diffuse responses. Successes and pitfalls with this method have been reviewed elsewhere (see Rapin, 1974).

Under no circumstances should screening audiometry be considered adequate for assessing children with delayed language. The authors insist that several hearing tests must be performed on each child before they can be satisfied that the test results are reliable.

Hearing impairment is even more likely to be misdiagnosed than total deafness. Hard of hearing children may become so adept at utilising their residual hearing and visual cues that they appear much less hearing impaired than they really are. High frequency hearing loss is particularly likely to be overlooked: the child with such impairment may respond to many environmental sounds, including language, at levels of normal or near normal intensity, but he develops little or no speech and fails to understand most of what is said to him. The low pitched components of language, including vowel sounds, carry little linguistic information. Consonants, which carry most of the linguistic information, are distinguished one from the other by transitions of high frequency components in the speech signal (Liberman *et al.*, 1967). Children with high frequency hearing losses (among them children who have suffered from kernicterus caused by neonatal hyperbilirubinaemia, most often secondary to blood group incompatibility) suffer from linguistic deprivation since discrimination of consonant sounds is difficult or impossible for them (Morley, 1972). Those with relatively mild deficits may simply substitute one consonant sound for another, or fail to produce specific speech sounds such as 's' and 'f'. The speech of children with severe hearing loss may be very poorly articulated or else articulation may be almost absent. Since the child is not deaf, he is likely to be mistaken for a child with primary language disability.

One should note that not all children with hearing impairments exhibit the behaviour one might expect of an intelligent deaf child: not all such children communicate eagerly and skilfully through non-acoustic channels, develop an elaborate system of gestures, attempt to lip-read, or appear normal in every respect except for linguistic behaviour. A few hearing impaired children develop autistic behaviour. Others are hyperactive and disorganised, especially in unstructured situations. They appear immature, usually because they have been overprotected and allowed little independence by their parents.

There is no clear answer as to how severe a hearing deficit has to be to account for the lack of language development. Some children, who have not had hearing aids or special education, are severely impaired with only moderate hearing losses (40–55 dB), while others, with greater losses, develop adequate speech, although with some deficits in articulation. That is, some hard of hearing children acquire language while others, who are equally impaired, do not; the reasons for this are still unclear. The nature of the hearing loss is an important factor. Children with flat hearing losses have the advantage over children with the same pure tone average but with a sloping threshold. One must consider the effect of environmental variables on language acquisition in children with hearing impairments. Age at which the hearing loss has been diagnosed, the child's linguistic environment, and adequacy of special education – all these factors must not be overlooked in assessing a child with hearing impairment who does not develop language skills as adequately as one might have expected.

If the child's hearing impairment in conjunction with his linguistic environment are judged insufficient to account for his language deficit, one must postulate the possibility that the child is also suffering from some form of brain dysfunction which is further interfering with his ability to learn language. Diseases which cause acquired hearing loss (intra- infection, hyperbilirubinaemia, neonatal anoxia, the complications of prematurity, purulent meningitis, etc.) often damage the brain, so that a hearing loss associated with brain dysfunction is not uncommon. But we stress that the brain dysfunction does not necessarily interact with the hearing loss. Some hearing impaired children with brain damage acquire language at precisely the same rate as hearing impaired children without brain damage. In the former cases it is assumed that the brain damage has spared the relevant neural systems.

DISORDERS OF AUDITORY PERCEPTION

Disorders of auditory perception in children have been studied in less detail than disorders of hearing and of linguistic processing. Discrimination of many features of auditory signals takes place at subcortical levels (Sachs, 1971). There is virtually no information about the effects of subcortical pathology on auditory perception in children, although it has been suggested that the auditory deficits of children who suffered from neonatal jaundice (kernicterus) (Carhart, 1967) and perhaps neonatal asphyxia (Hall, 1964) may reflect lesions in auditory relay nuclei in the brain stem. Sensitivity to intensity, pitch, onset and cessation of sound persists in animals who have had their auditory cortex ablated. In man, bilateral lesions of the primary auditory cortex do not produce deafness.

They may interfere with the recognition of environmental sounds and, invariably, with the ability to decode acoustically presented speech (Landau et al., 1960; Jerger et al., 1972; Goldstein, 1974; Chocholle et al., 1975). There is controversy to this time as to whether the deficit is in the perception of linguistic or auditory features. Unilateral lesions of the auditory cortex are difficult to demonstrate clinically and special tests are required in order to establish their presence (Lynn and Gilroy, 1972). Bocca et al. (1954) showed that the ability to perceive distorted speech and speech embedded in noise is deficient in the ear contralateral to a temporal lobe lesion. Heilman et al. (1973) proposed that this deficit is one of selective attention rather than of linguistic decoding. In patients with temporal lobe lesions, the perception of dichotic auditory stimuli (competing stimuli presented simultaneously to both ears) is also deficient in the ear contralateral to the lesion (Lowe et al., 1970). The work of Baru and Karaseva (1972) also points to the existence of a non-linguistic auditory deficit in such patients. They found that short acoustic stimuli have to be presented at higher intensities than longer ones in order to be perceived; an apparent deficit of temporal integration.

Non-linguistic auditory deficits have been described in some children with developmental language disability. A deficit in rate of auditory processing is suggested by the work of Lowe and Campbell (1965). They found that eight 'aphasoid' children required an interstimulus interval twice as long as normal children in order to be able to determine whether one or two tones had been presented. Tallal and Piercy (1973a) asked twelve children with developmental language disability to judge whether two successive tones were the same or different when frequency and interstimulus interval were varied. The results also showed that as interstimulus interval decreased, so did performance. Since these children had no difficulty with rapid visual sequences (Tallal and Piercy, 1973b), they concluded that the deficit was not one of rapid sensory processing in general, but that the cause of the children's language disability was a decreased rate of auditory processing. In contrast, Poppen et al. (1969) found that six children with language disability had difficulty in processing visual as well as auditory sequences. Aten and Davis (1968) have emphasised that difficulty with auditory memory and auditory sequences is not unique to children with language disability, but may be observed in children with brain damage but with normal language development. In their experiments the rate of presentation was not varied, and therefore they are not comparable to those of Lowe and Campbell (1965) and Tallal and Piercy (1973b). Another important point is that in most studies the performance of the language disabled children was not compared to that of children with brain damage but without language deficits. It is necessary to determine whether any of the deficits seen in children with language disability are specifically associated with the language defect or whether they reflect only the presence of brain damage.

The information on auditory perception in children with language disability is sparse and at present, not useful for clinical diagnosis. Furthermore, whether one can or indeed should differentiate between perception of non-linguistic auditory patterns and the decoding of acoustic speech remains controversial (Liberman *et al.*, 1967). This question however, will be discussed in detail by Tallal and Piercy in another chapter.

DISORDERS AFFECTING THE DECODING OF THE
PHONOLOGIC ASPECTS OF SPEECH
(VERBAL AUDITORY AGNOSIA)

These disorders must be clearly distinguished from global receptive language deficits. In children, global receptive deficits preclude the acquisition of language; verbal auditory agnosia however does not, providing that the input is not acoustic and the output is not speech (Stein and Curry, 1968; Worster-Drought, 1971). Verbal auditory agnosia (pure word deafness) was first recognised in adults who had sustained bilateral lesions involving the first temporal convolution; the lesions usually included Heschl's gyrus and adjacent auditory association cortex (Goldstein, 1974). The syndrome is rarely due to unilateral subcortical damage to the dominant side (Geschwind, 1965). A patient with pure word deafness stated: 'I can hear you talking, but I can't translate it'. (Jerger *et al.*, 1972). While these patients cannot repeat what has been said to them, they can express themselves verbally and their speech is normal or close to normal; although some have paraphasias, they do not speak in the jargon that is so characteristic of adults with receptive (Wernicke's) aphasia. They also remain able to read and write, while Wernicke's aphasics not. In verbal auditory agnosia, unlike Wernicke's aphasia, the deficit does not involve semantic processing. Linguistic processing is intact providing that the linguistic message is conveyed in a non-auditory code.

A child with a developmental language disability who came to autopsy suffered from lesions identical to those in adults with verbal auditory agnosia: he had cystic infarcts of both superior temporal convolutions and retrograde degeneration of the medial geniculate bodies (Landau *et al.*, 1960). The child was thought to have a hearing impairment in early life. Later, audiograms showed that hearing sensitivity was virtually normal, and it was apparent that the main deficit was an inability to comprehend spoken language. With special education, he learned to speak and understand speech, providing that each word was spoken slowly, and that there was a pause between them. The boy's lack of comprehension of acoustic speech when presented at a normal rate is consistent with the findings of

Tallal and Piercy (1973b), but there is no information as to whether he also had difficulty processing rapid non-linguistic acoustic sequences.

A syndrome of acquired verbal auditory agnosia in children has recently been discussed, and this may be relevant to the problem of developmental language disability. Several investigators, including Landau and Kleffner (1957), Stein and Curry (1968), Worster-Drought (1971), Gascon et. al. (1973), Rapin et al. (1977), among others, have described children with an acquired seizure disorder, characterised by short absences or staring attacks, associated with bilateral temporal EEG discharges. These children developed a severe receptive and expressive language deficit. Although previously their language development had been normal, they became mute and unable to process acoustic language. Some learned the sign language of the deaf and reading and writing, but only when this was taught with methods appropriate for deaf children (Stein and Curry, 1968; Worster-Drought, 1971). The fact they learned to read indicates that they were not suffering from a global language disability. Rather, their deficits, like those of adults with pure word deafness, were restricted to the decoding of acoustic speech. Their inability to speak is interpreted as secondary to the receptive deficit and analogous to the almost immediate loss of speech experienced by normal children who, in early childhood, suddenly lose their hearing.

It seems likely that at least some children with developmental language disability have essentially the same problem as those with acquired verbal auditory agnosia, Rapin et al. (1977) investigated two brothers with a severe receptive deficit for acoustic language: the older boy had staring spells and developed an auditory agnosia between the ages of 2 and 3 years – after he had acquired his language; his younger brother, on the other hand, never spoke normally, had no seizures, and had a normal EEG. The brothers' linguistic problems appeared similar, but one presented the clinical picture of an acquired verbal auditory agnosia, the other a developmental language disability. Another boy, who lost his speech at 3 years of age, had the characteristic EEG described above, but without seizures. Yet another, one of 24 children with developmental language disability, who never spoke (Rapin et al., unpublished), also had bilateral EEG discharges but no seizures, and Goldstein et al. (1960) have reported that EEG abnormalities without clinical seizures are common in children with developmental language disability. These observations highlight the need to obtain an EEG in all children with developmental dysphasia, even when there is no clinical evidence of seizures. They also indicate that some children with developmental language disability have a syndrome which appears to be closely related to that seen in children with verbal auditory agnosia.

Disorders of Linguistic Processing

Knowledge of the brain functions which underlie central linguistic processing in children is sparse. Most of what we know is based on extrapolation from adult aphasics. The extent to which similar processes are involved in normal language acquisition is unknown.

DISORDERS OF LANGUAGE AND CEREBRAL SPECIALISATION (HEMISPHERIC ASYMMETRY)

The processing of language engages left hemispheric activity in virtually all right-handed, and in many left-handed and ambidextrous individuals. Anatomic differences between the two temporal lobes are present at birth (Witelson and Pallie, 1973; Wada et al., 1975). Also experiments with dichotic presentation of auditory stimuli suggest specialisation of the left hemisphere for language processing from early childhood (Kimura, 1963; Lowe et al., 1970; Ingram, 1975). There is, however, other evidence which suggests that language engages the activity of both hemispheres to a greater extent in young children than in mature individuals; unilateral brain lesions sustained in early life and severe enough to produce hemiplegia, whether they affect the left or the right hemisphere, do not preclude language acquisition (Basser, 1962; Annett, 1973); removal of the hemisphere contralateral to an infantile hemiplegia, whether it be the right or the left, does not interfere with language (Basser, 1962); and recovery from acquired aphasia in children occurs in almost all cases and quite rapidly, providing that the child has not suffered from severe bilateral damage.

Because unilateral brain damage has not been demonstrated to interfere with language acquisition, regardless of the laterality of lesion, it was assumed that developmental language disability was unlikely to be the consequence of focal damage to the left hemisphere. Recent radiographic evidence suggests that this may not be so: of 87 pneumoencephalograms in children with developmental language disability suspected of structural brain damage, 26 showed enlargement of the left temporal horn, 6 of the right, and 14 of both temporal horns. In contrast, of 79 pneumoencephalograms of children with petit mal epilepsy and no linguistic impairment, 6 showed enlargement of the left, 5 of the right, and 6 of both lateral ventricles (Dalby, 1975). In another study, 15 of 17 'autistic' children who failed to acquire expressive language and had impaired receptive skills were found to have dilated left ventricles, and particularly enlargement of the left temporal horn (Hauser et al., 1975). If one views autism as a syndrome in which severe or total failure of communication and gross derangement of affect are salient features, these findings will not come as a total surprise. Medial temporal structures are part of the limbic system which plays a central role in learning and in the elaboration of drives and emotions. The lateral temporal cortex is concerned with auditory and, in the left hemisphere, with linguistic processing. While such an explanation is undoubtedly simplistic and can by no means account for all the manifestations of the autistic syndrome or of developmental language disability, these radiographic observations do suggest that further research is necessary to delineate the syndromes of brain dysfunction in non-verbal children.

The child neurologist who studies developmental language disability will not encounter the relatively clear syndromes seen in adult aphasics (Marin *et al.* (1976), Geschwind, 1971). Even acquired aphasia tends to affect language less selectively in children than in adults: fluent aphasia do not occur, perhaps because language is not yet an overlearned skill requiring little monitoring (Geschwind, 1968); most children with an acquired aphasia are initially mute, regardless of the area of greatest pathology (Alajouanine and Lhermitte, 1965). Most recover rapidly, perhaps because the right hemisphere becomes available or regains the capacity to mediate the processing of language and the programming of speech.

SYNDROMES IN CHILDREN WITH DEFICIENT LANGUAGE DEVELOPMENT

Rapin *et al.* and Wilson *et al.* (unpublished) having collected linguistic, neuropsychological and neurological data from approximately 60 preschool and school-age children with language disabilities receiving remedial education found that the children differ from one another in their ability to comprehend, speak spontaneously and in structured interchanges, and also in their ability to repeat verbal utterances. The children varied in their semantic, syntactical, and phonological skills. Most of the children had oral-motor deficits and were delayed in achieving motor milestones such as walking. Deficits of fine motor abilities, while present in fewer children, tended to persist into school age. Some children had no deficits in memory, perception, or cognition when the stimuli are presented in the visual modality, but they show conspicuous deficits in analogous tasks when the stimuli are presented in the auditory modality. Other children who show a significant difficulty with visually presented tasks show no difficulty with the auditory perception of linguistic and non-linguistic stimuli and no deficit of memory for sequential and non-sequential auditory stimuli, while comprehension of language presented acou tically is severely impaired. Such children appear deficient in the semantic aspects of language, while syntax and phonology are relatively unaffected. The performance of some children improves when stimuli are presented in the auditory and visual modalities simultaneously, while the performance of others deteriorates markedly. The therapeutic 'multisensory stimulation' approach suggested by Fernald (1943) and Gillingham and Sillman (1956) is clearly of questionable value with this latter group.

The clustering of deficits along various linguistic and neuropsychological dimensions suggests that it will be possible to define syndromes of disability in children with developmental language impairment. We will give descriptions of children with particularly salient characteristics in order to illustrate some of the syndromes we are attempting to define.

We have seen a 4-year-old girl whose spontaneous verbalisations were syntactically, semantically and phonologically impeccable but often unrelated to the situation in which she found herself and to the questions put to her. She had a severe deficit of short-term auditory memory, but functioned at levels appropriate for her age if the stimuli were presented to the visual modality. She had no motor deficits but did have difficulty with spatial-constructional and graphomotor tasks. In another case, a boy of superior intelligence spoke in unintelligible jargon at 5 years of age. When he was 8 years old he spoke fluently, and his only deficits were in synthesising words and nonsense syllables from discretely presented phonemes, adding a phoneme to complete a word, and providing inflections for various parts of speech ('Sound Blending, Auditory Closure, and Grammatic Closure subtests of the ITPA'. Kirk et al., 1968). A third subject, a $4\frac{1}{2}$-year-old boy with severe oral-motor apraxia, and syntactic and word finding difficulty scored at the 90th percentile in cognitive, linguistic and perceptual tests, so long as the response required was not a verbal one. He had no difficulty with the comprehension of acoustic language. Finally, a 9-year-old boy with deficits in oral-motor, oculomotor and fine motor coordination had profound syntactic, semantic, and phonological difficulties. He had restricted spontaneous speech. His deficits included comprehension, spontaneous speech and repetition. In addition, he had widespread impairment in non-linguistic areas, including perception and memory for haptic, acoustic and visual stimuli. He had no graphomotor or spatial-constructional deficits.

At present we have few clues as to the cause and localisation of cerebral dysfunction in these children. On the basis of their clinical history and the findings on neurological examination, a few of them are thought to have sustained brain lesions in early life. In the majority, we are not yet in a position to differentiate between a developmental (genetic?) and an acquired syndrome. We are currently attempting to delineate profiles of deficits in the children we have studied along neurological, neuropsychological and linguistic dimensions, whilst Aram and Nation (1975) have developed linguistic profiles based on the children's performance on semantic, syntactic, and phonological dimensions on the basis of their spontaneous speech, repetition, and comprehension.

Our results do not support the notion that a single deficit is likely to be found in all children with developmental language disorders. Eisenson (1972) and Tallal and Piercy (1973a) see difficulty with the processing of sequential auditory stimuli as a primary cause in virtually all children with developmental language disability. Others emphasise expressive deficits: Menyuk (1964) and Kerschensteiner and Huber (1975) stress defective syntax, poor articulation, and an impoverished vocabulary; while in Morley's (1972) experience, children with severely retarded language development are much more likely to have expressive than receptive deficits.

LANGUAGE DISORDERS: THE ROLE OF SHORT-TERM AUDITORY MEMORY

Short-term auditory memory plays a crucial role in verbal comprehension. The work of Conrad (1972), in particular, indicates that verbal stimuli pass into an acoustic short-term store where phonological, syntactic and semantic operations are carried out in order to extract their meaning. Lesions involving the supramarginal and angular gyri of the left parietal lobe profoundly interfere with short-term verbal acoustic memory, at least in adults, and produce an amnestic aphasia (word finding difficulty) (Geschwind, 1967; Warrington et al., 1971). Fedio (1976) was able to interfere selectively with registration and retrieval of verbal labels, depending on whether he stimulated the left temporal cortex anteriorly or posteriorly, during surgical procedures for the control of epilepsy.

Some children with developmental language disability may have particular difficulty with certain but not all types of auditory sequences: nonverbal acoustic signals, nonsense syllables, words, or sentences. The same may be said for visual memory. When the two sensory modalities are combined, performance improves in some children but deteriorates in others. We are still attempting to elaborate the nature of the interaction, but as yet we have no predictive indices. A battery of tests of acoustic, visual, and combined auditory-visual memory are therefore included in the neuropsychological investigation of children with developmental language disability.

General Disorders of Brain Function which may Affect Language Acquisition

HYPERKINETIC SYNDROME

Children who fail to develop an appropriate level of verbal communication are frequently distractible and disorganised. While the hyperkinetic syndrome is, undoubtedly, detrimental to language acquisition, especially in a child for whom successful communication requires particular effort, it is doubtful that hyperkinesis alone is the cause of the language disability. Distractability can be reduced in some children by providing a structured environment and reinforcing attentive behaviour, while others would benefit from pharmacological control.

AUTISM

Autism was touched upon earlier. While most children with developmental language disability are not autistic, young autistic children have profoundly disordered verbal communication. They are often mute or echolalic (Rutter, 1971). The authors agree with those workers who view autism as a consequence of severe derangement of brain function and almost never as the consequence of environmental or affective deprivation (Rutter, 1971; DeMyer et al., 1973; Hauser et al., 1975). Although many autistic children have no language, they tend to be more severely lacking in symbolic behaviour than children with developmental language disability who do not have autistic features; their play, for instance is unimaginative, and most do not develop a gesture language. The long-term outlook for autistic children is very poor, even with massive educational efforts and parental counselling (DeMyer et al., 1975).

DEFICITS OF COGNITIVE COMPETENCE

Mental retardation may be defined as an impairment which affects all areas of behaviour, although not necessarily to the same extent. As one would expect, the linguistic skills of retarded children tend to be less advanced than those of normal children, especially during early childhood. Lenneberg (1967), among others, has pointed out that language acquisition in the retarded child proceeds until early adolescence when it reaches an asymptote. The acquisition of the most important syntactical and phonological rules is well advanced by about the age of 4 in normal children. Retarded children with a mental age above 4 years can be expected to have adequate linguistic skills. Only profoundly retarded children remain essentially non-verbal. The small proportion of moderately retarded children whose linguistic skills are significantly below their levels of attainment in other areas must therefore be looked upon as both mentally retarded and language-impaired.

Children with primary language disability may appear to be mentally retarded (i.e. to have a general cognitive impairment) if tested inappropriately. For instance, the ubiquitous Stanford-Binet test, which remains a favoured psychometric instrument for testing young children, gives the least valid measure of cognitive competence in children with language disability. The test is so constructed that it is not possible to segregate 'verbal' from 'performance' levels; also, given skills cannot be assessed along developmental continua. After the age of 3, the test is heavily loaded with language items, both auditory and visual, and therefore is particularly unsuitable for children with language disability. In fact, some language disordered children whose test scores on the Stanford-Binet Scale indicates the presence of mental retardation, when tested with non-verbal tests such as the Hiskey-Nebraska Test of Learning Aptitude (Hiskey, 1955) or the Pictorial Test of Intelligence (French, 1964) show an intellectual ability within or above the normal range. Physicians and educators themselves must learn to evaluate the psychometric test used in assessing these children before they accept summary scores such as IQ figures, as they may reflect neither their deficient verbal ability nor their perhaps quite adequate non-verbal skills.

Disorders of Speech Output

DEFECTIVE PHONEMIC AND SYNTACTIC PROGRAMMING

Children with this type of difficulty produce speech which may be almost unintelligible to all but close members of their family. These children appear to understand what is said to them, although discrimination of speech sounds is usually somewhat impaired, and comprehension is below expected levels. Analysis of the children's utterances shows not only mispronunciations (distortions, inversions, substitutions involving consonants, especially consonant clusters, and syllables), but also syntactic errors and aberrant word order (Shriner *et al.*, 1969). As in the adult with expressive aphasia, small words (articles, prepositions, pronouns) are likely to be missing. Speech may be 'primitive', consisting mainly of one or two word utterances, usually nouns and uninflected verbs, resembling the speech of a younger child. Some of these children may have an oral-motor apraxia and pseudobulbar signs, but these are viewed as added symptoms to a linguistic deficit. In a number of these children, as in those with a purely phonemic difficulty, prognosis tends to be good. It is likely that in some children, notably those without dysarthria, the syndrome may represent a developmental delay and in some cases have a genetic aetiology. Prognosis is not always favourable, however, since we have observed persistent and significant deficits even in pre-adolescents. Criteria for differentiating between pathological language development and delayed acquisition of language in pre-school children are not yet available. Speech which remains grossly abnormal by the time the child reaches school age can be accepted as prime evidence for cerebral pathology.

DEFECTIVE PHONEMIC PROGRAMMING

It is not certain whether it is legitimate to separate this syndrome from the one discussed previously, as it may represent only a milder variant. Syntax is intact but phonological programming is inadequate (Yoss and Darley, 1974). Some of these children may represent no more than a subgroup at the extreme of phonemic immaturity which characterises so many otherwise normal pre-school children. Prognosis is nearly always good, although some abnormal speech sounds may persist into adult language.

DYSARTHRIA

This term is being used to indicate a non-linguistic motor deficit of the speech mechanisms. These deficits may involve the supranuclear control of the muscles of articulation by corticobulbar fibres and the pathways from the cerebellum and basal ganglia. In other cases, the lower motor neurons, the myoneural junction, or the muscles themselves may be affected. In all of these disorders, the motor deficit will involve not only speech, but also swallowing, sucking, whistling, phonation and, in some cases, breathing. The neurologist must seek to distinguish among these causes of dysarthria in his attempt to localise the site of pathology and its aetiology.

Pseudobulbar palsy, due to a lesion of the upper motor neurons projecting on to the lower cranial nerve nuclei (corticobulbar pathway), will be manifested by spasticity of the facial and oropharyngeal muscles and hyperactive reflexes such as the jaw jerk, facial reflexes and gag reflex (Illingworth, 1969). The child will have difficulty controlling individual muscles, and complex motor sequences such as swallowing and articulation will be deficient. In severe cases children may be unable to move the tongue or shape the lips imitatively. They often have relatively inexpressive faces and are likely to drool excessively.

Lesions involving the basal ganglia, the most common manifestation of which is athetoid cerebral palsy, produce abnormal involuntary movements, facial grimacing, tongue thrusting, irregular respiration, and, again, interruption and uncoordination of complex motor sequences. Articulation is defective, voicing is poorly modulated, rhythm is markedly slowed down, and speech is often nasal. In some infants, chewing and swallowing may be so severely affected as to necessitate gavage feeding.

Disorders of supranuclear control of speech are frequently associated with an oral-motor apraxia: the child may have difficulty making certain movements with his tongue, lips or jaw to verbal command, or in imitation of the examiner, but he can produce the same movement as part of a spontaneous motor sequence (Kools *et al.*, 1971). For instance, he fails to open and close his jaw when requested to do so, but is able to yawn; he cannot protrude his tongue on command, but will lick his lips while eating. Oral-motor apraxias are common in children with pathology of the corticobulbar and basal ganglia pathways. They are also common in children with speech difficulties in whom linguistic and non-linguistic deficits usually coincide. Oral-motor apraxia can be viewed as a disorder of programming which is not specific to speech movements but involves simpler motor sequences as well.

Cerebellar disturbances of speech, which are very rare in young children, mostly interfere with speech rhythm; they are more common in older children and adults with acquired diffuse lesions of the cerebellum. In these children speech is scanning i.e. segments of speech are accelerated and separated by pauses which do not necessarily coincide with the pauses of normal speech. Respiration is often irregular. In advanced cases of cerebellar disturbance coordination may become so poor that there is interference with the production of individual speech sounds, and, in extreme cases, anarthria may result.

In bulbar palsy, lesions affect the nuclei of the cranial nerves in the brain stem. Children with congenital facial palsy have difficulty sucking in infancy and, later, in articulating labials. In diseases with extensive involvement of lower cranial nerve nuclei, all motor functions of the face, mouth, pharynx, and larynx may be affected. Bulbar palsy is characterised by flaccid paralysis with areflexia. Nasal voice, hypophonia, regurgitation of fluid through the nose, weakness of the tongue, and pooling of oral secretions are among its characteristic features. The neurologist will also note loss of the gag reflex, fasciculation of the tongue, atrophy of the involved muscles, and weakness of the cough because of inability to close the glottis, often associated with weakness of chest muscles.

STUTTERING

This disorder is mentioned here because it is viewed as a disorder in the programming of speech output. Theories as to its cause are controversial (Morley, 1972) and range from emotional disturbance, to the learning of a maladaptive pattern of speech, to a developmental lag, or to a neurological disturbance perhaps involving competition between outputs from the two hemispheres seeking to gain access to the brain stem nuclei which constitute the final common pathway for the production of speech (Jones, 1966). Child neurologists are rarely required to examine stuttering children since most stutterers have no other evidence of neurological dysfunction, and since their language, as opposed to their speech, is usually normal. It may be worth noting that speech disturbances which are very similar to or actually share many aspects with idiopathic stuttering are encountered in some progressive diffuse diseases of the brain, in particular juvenile cerebromacular degeneration, where they are thought to reflect pathology in the basal ganglia (Schain and Wiley, 1965).

Neurological Investigation of the Child with a Developmental Language Disability

The tools which the neurologist has at his disposal include the clinical history, physical, neurological and developmental assessments, audiological evaluation, and the results of laboratory studies.

It is beyond the scope of this chapter to describe in detail the ways in which a neurological examination in an infant or a small child should be carried out; this has been described in detail in several reviews (Peiper, 1963; Illingworth, 1966; Dekaban, 1970; Ingram and Henderson, 1972) and will not be reiterated here. It is, however, important to bear in mind the limitations of the information which can be collected in the assessment of a very young child.

The point of the preceding sections was to discuss the types of information the child neurologist is trying to discover. As he speaks to the parents and examines the child, he has in mind a schema of the oral-aural system. As stated in the introduction, his aim is on the one hand to seek evidence for dysfunction(s) at each level of this system and, on the other, to ask himself what cause(s) he can discover to explain the observed dysfunction(s).

Unfortunately, there will be only few cases in which he will provide a definite answer to the two problems of localisation and cause of cerebral dysfunction. Most of the time multiple dysfunctions will be found and several possible explanations, or none at all, uncovered. Several new questions will have to be faced. The physician will have to decide whether all these dysfunctions fit together into a coherent syndrome. For instance, hyperbilirubinaemia in an infant may produce a hearing loss, paralysis of upward gaze and choreoathetosis. These disparate findings, pointing to multiple areas of dysfunction in the brain and resulting in multiple handicaps for the child, can be the result of a single insult to the immature nervous system. Language and speech are defective because of an input disorder (high frequency loss) and output disorder (choreoathetosis). If the hyperbilirubinaemia occurred in a premature infant who sustained anoxic episodes, the examination may also reveal spasticity and microcephaly. Such a child may have pseudobulbar palsy and oral-motor apraxia in addition to choreoathetosis; he may also be mentally retarded. In attempting to discover why such a child lacks speech, the neurologist will have to weigh the contributions of each dysfunction to each of the deficits in the communication system. Perhaps lack of speech is the result of lack of comprehension: is lack of comprehension attributable to hearing loss, or to cognitive incompetence, or both? Or, perhaps, comprehension of oral speech, although not perfect, is adequate for the acquisition of language: in this case, lack of speech may be the consequence of pseudobulbar palsy or athetosis.

The average non-verbal child whom the child neurologist is asked to examine does not usually have such gross evidence of neurological impairment, and evidence from his clinical history will be less clear-cut. The history may reveal that the child's parents are not English speaking, that their socio-economic circumstances are poor, and that they have a limited education. The gestation was said to be marred by moderate toxaemia in the last month of pregnancy, delivery was induced, his birth weight low for gestational age, but no catastrophes were known to have taken place in the neonatal period. Records of the child's birth are unavailable, or if obtained, contain so little information as to be useless. Details of illness in infancy are not recalled, the child was hospitalised once for pneumonia and diarrhoea (or was it croup, or meningitis?). He walked at about 18 months and now, at 30 months, he is saying only 'mama' and 'dada'. General physical examination is unrevealing except that the child's height and weight are at the third percentile for age and his head circumference just below the third percentile. Neurological examination is frustratingly incomplete, because the child clings to his mother and engages in little play. His gait appears normal, his eye movements and facial movements are normal, he does not drool (but sucks on a pacifier throughout the examination). He pushes away blocks or toys offered to him without evidence of dysmetria. He does not exhibit abnormal involuntary movements. He looks at the examiner, shyly lifting his head from his mother's lap. He is silent except that he cries when an attempt is made to test his reflexes, look in his eyes, or detach him from his mother.

Or perhaps a slightly older child walks into the office and proceeds to explore it, ignoring the examiner and his mother. He plays with the water, splashing the floor and soaking himself, tears up paper offered to him to write on, pushes down the towers of blocks the examiner makes in an attempt to engage him in constructive play, fiddles with the blood pressure cuff, opens drawers and rifles their contents, and appears quite content as long as no demands are made on him. He pulls away or screams when the examiner attempts to direct his activities. Again, gait, coordination, eye and face movements are normal. Can he hear? Can't he or won't he pile blocks, draw a line, obey verbal commands? Is he retarded, hearing impaired, autistic, or is his main problem a developmental language disability?

Such stories, so often repeated in the child neurologist's office, are offered here to indicate the limitations of his evaluation. Even though he obtains a family tree and detailed history of pregnancy, birth, neonatal events, and intercurrent illnesses, certain events in his clinical history must be looked upon as possible, but not definite, causes of his language retardation. And even though the neurologist has trained himself to observe rather than manipulate, and has developed ingenious tricks to elicit information about gross and fine motor coordination, eye movements, face and tongue movements, attention, spatial skills, etc., his evaluation will necessarily be gross, qualitative and tentative. His evaluation of the clinical history will provide possible risk factors more often than definite aetiologies.

The child neurologist's evaluation frequently does not provide enough information to arrive at a precise diagnosis. While records of the child's medical history are hopefully complete, his findings on examination can only serve as pointers towards more detailed investigations to be carried out by others.

What laboratory tests does he have at his disposal? Microscopical and biochemical tests of blood and urine will only be useful in the very rare cases when he is looking for a specific syndrome, such as a metabolic disease, or immunological evidence for an intra-uterine infection. Chromosome analysis is almost never fruitful even in clearly genetic cases, except in children in whom obviously abnormal features are found on physical examination. Radiographs of the skull are rarely useful. There are almost no cases where invasive procedures, such as pneumoencephalography and cerebral angiography, are justified. On the other hand, the advent of the non-invasive computerised transaxial tomography scan (CTT) affords new possibilities for defining the frequency and types of structural brain lesions found in children who fail to develop language. The previously described studies of Hauser et al. (1975) and Dalby (1975) suggest that the proportion of gross lesions may be higher than suspected. This knowledge will be very valuable from a theoretical standpoint, and useful both for the parents of the child and the professionals who work with them. Those children who do not speak and appear autistic and are found to have gross lesions of the brain, need no longer be regarded as 'emotionally disturbed', and other hypotheses have to be offered to explain their deficits (Hauser *et al.*, 1975). It will be possible to compare non-verbal children both with and without brain lesions in terms of behavioural assessment and linguistic performance, which will add further to the delineation of syndromes.

An electroencephalogram (EEG) should be obtained in children who do not speak. A normal EEG does not, of course, rule out brain dysfunction. Mild and diffuse EEG abnormalities may provide no help, since such abnormalities are non-specific and found in a proportion of normal children. It is important to be aware that the interpretation of EEG records in young children is fraught with possibilities for error, since the EEG changes drastically with cerebral maturation. Many young children must be sedated in order to make EEG recording possible. Sleep itself introduces changes in the EEG which varies with the stage or depth of sleep, and some sedatives modify background rhythms. Even experienced electroencephalographers may never reach complete agreement on the interpretation of children's records. In our experience, electroencephalographers who only occasionally read children's records are prone to overread them and report significant changes which others would regard as normal variants. Despite these drawbacks, and the fact that most non-verbal children do not have significant EEG abnormalities, this test is considered important because the discovery of a frank EEG focus, especially in temporal or temporo-parietal regions, is highly significant. The discovery of bilateral paroxysmal EEG discharges is crucial since it may indicate that the cause of the language abnormality is a verbal auditory agnosia and that anticonvulsant drugs should be prescribed, although with no guarantee that they will affect the child's course significantly.

Finally, the child neurologist must refer every child who does not speak or whose speech is significantly abnormal for a detailed and competent audiological investigation. The terms 'detailed' and 'competent' are stressed since the difficulties and pitfalls of this investigation are great, and since the statistical probability of finding a hearing problem in a child who fails to develop language is high. We again stress the need for repeated testing, even if the original results appear reliable, since, in our experience, errors in estimating threshold occur even with multiple tests and independent assessments (Rapin and Costa, 1969). Tests should be repeated over many months, or even several years, until there is no doubt in anyone's mind that the results are accurate and valid.

Integration of the Neurologist's Findings with those of Other Professionals

The results of the neurologist's investigation will usually be made available to psychologists, audiologists, speech pathologists, and possibly linguists who will also evaluate the child. While the other professionals may elicit further details to enlarge the clinical history, the core of their investigation will be a detailed and, hopefully, quantitative investigation of the child's linguistic and adaptive behaviour. The role of the neurologist can be looked upon as a coarse screen for many aspects of sensory-motor and adaptive behaviour, enabling others to focus in greater detail upon areas where dysfunction was detected. True, each professional in turn assesses and then focuses on promising areas, but the neurologist's screening, while less refined in many ways, is likely to provide broader information than that of other professionals: he knows less about more.

When the other professionals have evaluated the child, and the results of laboratory investigations have become available, it is essential that all those involved in the case should meet and discuss the child. This will provide a chance to discover areas of agreement and disagreement among the assessors, and to highlight aspects of behaviour which no one alone has succeeded in obtaining because of possible lack of cooperation or inability of the child to produce such behaviour. A tentative description regarding areas of deficient as well as adequate function should be outlined. Possible or probable causes of the dysfunction need to be considered. Recommendations for a detailed and specific educational programme must be drawn up and a timetable for future follow-up agreed upon.

At this stage, one person who should be in charge of the case must be selected. In practice, this is usually the child's paediatrician or family physician. If he is to play this role, he must participate actively in the evaluation conference. Others, however, may take charge of the case, for instance the child neurologist, the psychologist, the speech pathologist, or the social worker. The person in charge must be familiar with the type of disability shown by the child and with the educational and remedial resources available for treatment. If he is to be effective, all communications concerning the child's case must be directed to him. In turn, he must be responsible to the parents for the interpretation of the case and also in ensuring that the recommendations made by those involved are implemented.

Finally, these efforts are wasted unless the findings and recommendations are communicated clearly and succinctly to the parents, and unless the parents are given an opportunity to ask the questions which, undoubtedly, will have come to their minds as their child is investigated. While the person in charge of the case should lead the informing interview, it is essential that a physician should participate in order to answer questions about medical causes. The physician will often be the child's neurologist, since his training enables him to take a broad view of the problem. The number and type of professionals involved in the case depend on the child's specific problem and its particular complexities.

Need for Longitudinal Follow-up

At the end of the lengthy initial evaluation, a definitive diagnosis may still remain elusive. We emphasise that therapy and the start of special education should not await a definitive diagnosis but that both should be started as soon as the areas of greatest deficiency have been identified. When in doubt, it is preferable to carry on with remedial training and allow sufficient time to elapse before evaluating results. The need for a long-term assessment is implicit in this approach.

Another point worth stressing is that the educator's or therapist's experience with the child and the child's response to remediation may provide the most valuable and valid estimate of his strengths and deficits. The diagnosis will often be much more obvious in a child who has become used to interacting with adults other than those in his immediate family. A child who could not be adequately examined on first interview may now be cooperative and eager to perform.

The child neurologist, as well as other professionals, must see the child more than once in order to evaluate developmental progress and the effects of remediation, and to refine and revise his assessment of areas of neurological dysfunction. This reassessment means that errors in diagnosis can be corrected and also that an incomplete initial evaluation can be concluded. The neurologist needs to know of any development in the child's case, so that he can learn about the outcome of these disorders and also compare and contrast different clinical histories. In this way he can become more effective in dealing with future cases.

Acknowledgements

Supported in part by grants NS3356 and 2T1 NS5325 from the National Institute of Neurological Diseases, Communication Disorders and Stroke, United States Public Health Service, and grant OEG 0-74-0545 from the Bureau of Education for the Handicapped, Office of Education, Department of Health, Education and Welfare.

References

Alajouanine, T. and Lhermitte, F. (1965). Acquired aphasia in children. *Brain* **88**, 653–662.

Annett, M. (1973). Laterality of childhood hemiplegia and the growth of speech and intelligence. *Cortex* **9**, 4–29.

Aram, D. M. and Nation, J. E. (1975). Patterns of language behavior in children with developmental language disorders. *J. Speech Hear. Res.* **18**, 229–241.

Aten, J. and Davis, J. (1968). Disturbances in the perception of auditory sequence in children with minimal cerebral dysfunction. *J. Speech. Hear. Res.* **11**, 236–245.

Barr, B. (1955). Pure tone audiometry for preschool children. *Acta oto-lar.*, Suppl. **121**, 1–84.

Baru, A. V. and Karaseva, T. A. (1972). 'The Brain and Hearing. Hearing Disturbances Associated with Local Brain Lesions'. Consultants Bureau, New York and London.

Basser, L. S. (1962). Hemipiegia of early onset and the faculty of speech with special reference to the effects of hemispherectomy. *Brain* **85**, 427–460.

Bocca, E., Callaro, C. and Cassinari, V. (1954). A new method for testing hearing in temporal lobe tumors, preliminary report. *Acta oto-lar.* **44**, 219–221.

Carhart, R. (1967). Probable mechanisms underlying kernicteric hearing loss. *Acta oto-lar.*, Suppl. **221**, 1–41.

Chocholle, R., Chedru, F., Botte, M. C. *et al.* (1975). Etude psychoacoustique d'un cas de 'surdité corticale'. *Neuropsychologia* **13**, 163–172.

Conrad, R. (1972). The developmental role of vocalizing in short-term memory. *J. Verbal Learn. Verbal Behav.* **11**, 521–533.

Crowley, D. E., Davis, H. and Beagley, H. A. (1975). Survey of the clinical use of electrocochleography. *Ann. Otol. Rhin. Laryngol.* (St Louis) **84**, 297–307.

Dalby, M. A. (1975). 'Air Studies in Language-Retarded Children. Evidence of Early Lateralization of Language Function'. Presented at 1st International Congress of Child Neurology, Toronto, October 1975.

Dekaban, A. (1970). 'Neurology of Early Childhood', Ch. 2, pp. 50–81. Williams and Wilkins Co., Baltimore.

DeMyer, M. K. (1975). The nature of the neuropsychological disability in autistic children. *J. Autism Child. Schizophr.* **5**, 109–128.

DeMyer, M. K., Barton, S., DeMyer, W. E. *et al.* (1973). Prognosis in autism: A follow-up study. *J. Autism Child. Schizophr.* **3**, 199–246.

Dix, M. R. and Hallpike, C. S. (1947). Peepshow: New technique for pure tone audiometry in young children. *Brit. Med. J.* **2**, 719–723.

Eisenson, J. (1972). 'Aphasia in Children'. Harper and Row, New York.

Fedio, P. (1976). 'The Cortical and Thalamic Mechanisms of Memory'. Presented at the International Neuropsychology Society Annual Meeting, Toronto, February, 1976.

Fernald, G. M. (1943). 'Remedial Techniques in Basic School Subjects'. McGraw-Hill, New York.

French, J. L. (1964). 'Pictorial Test of Intelligence'. Houghton Mifflin, New York.

Gascon, G., Victor, D., Lombroso, C. T. and Goodglass, H. (1973). Language disorder, convulsive disorder and electroencephalographic abnormalities. *Arch. Neurol.* **28**, 156–162.

Geschwind, N. (1965). Disconnexion syndromes in animals and man. *Brain* **88**, 237–294 and 585–644.

Geschwind, N. (1967). The varieties of naming errors. *Cortex* **3**, 97–112.

Geschwind, N. (1968). Neurologic Foundations of Language. *In* 'Progress in Learning Disabilities' (H. R. Myklebust, ed.), pp. 182–198. Grune and Stratton, New York.

Geschwind, N. (1971). Aphasia. *New Engl. J. Med.* **284**, 654–657.

Gillingham, A. and Stillman, B. (1956). 'Remedial Reading Training for Children with Specific Disabilities in Reading, Spelling and Penmanship'. Bronxville, New York.

Goldstein, M. N. (1974). Auditory agnosia for speech ('Pure word-deafness'). *Brain Lang.* **1**, 195–204.

Goldstein, R., Landau, W. M. amd Kleffner, F. R. (1960). Neurologic observations in a population of deaf and aphasic children. *Ann. Otol.* **69**, 756–768.

Hall, J. (1964). On the neuropathological changes in the central nervous system following neonatal asphyxia with special reference to the auditory system in man. *Acta oto-lar.* Suppl. **188**, 331–338.

Hauser, S. L., DeLong, R. and Rosman, N. P. (1975). Pneumographic findings in the infantile autism syndrome: A correlation with temporal lobe disease. *Brain* **98**, 667–688.

Heilman, K. M., Hammer, L. C. and Wilder, B. J. (1973). An audiometric defect in temporal lobe dysfunction. *Neurology* **23**, 384–386.

Hiskey, M. S. (1955). The Hiskey-Nebraska Test for Learning Aptitude. (Rev.) University of Nebraska, Lincoln.

Illingworth, R. S. (1966). 'The Development of the Infant and Young Child; Normal and Abnormal', 3rd edition. E. and S. Livingstone Ltd, Edinburgh.

Illingworth, R. S. (1969). Sucking and swallowing difficulties in infancy: Diagnostic problem of dysphagia. *Arch. Dis. Childh.* **44**, 655–665.

Ingram, D. (1975). Cerebral speech lateralization in young children. *Neuropsychologia* **13**, 103–105.

Ingram, T. T. S. (1959). Specific developmental disorder of speech in childhood. *Brain* **82**, 450–467.

Ingram, T. T. S. and Henderson, A. (1972). The Assessment of a Child in a Special Clinic. *In* 'The Child with Delayed Speech' (M. Rutter and J. A. M. Martin, eds), pp. 68–82, Clinics in Developmental Medicine No. 43, Spastics International Medical Publications. Heinemann Medical Books Ltd, London. J. B. Lippincott Co., Philadelphia.

Jerger, J., Lovering, L. and Wertz, M. (1972). Auditory disorder following bilateral temporal lobe insult: Report of a case. *J. Speech Hear. Dis.* **37**, 523–535.

Jones, R. K. (1966). Observations on stammering after localized cerebral injury. *J. Neurol. Neurosurg. Psychiat.* **29**, 192–195.

Kerschensteiner, M. and Huber, W. (1975). Grammatical impairment in developmental aphasia. *Cortex* 11, 264–282.

Kimura, D. (1963). Speech lateralization in young children as determined by an auditory test. *J. Comp. Physiol. Psychol.* 56, 899–902.

Kirk, S. A., McCarthy, J. J. and Kirk, W. D. (1968). 'Illinois Test of Psycholinguistic Abilities'. University of Illinois Press, Urbana.

Kools, J. A., Williams, A. F., Vickers, M. J. and Caell, A. (1971). Oral and limb apraxia in mentally retarded children with deviant articulation. *Cortex* 7, 387–400.

Landau, W. M., Goldstein, R. and Kleffner, E. R. (1960). Congenital aphasia: A clinicopathologic study. *Neurology* 10, 915–921.

Landau, W. M. and Kleffner, F. R. (1957). Syndrome of acquired aphasia with convulsive disorder in children. *Neurology* 7, 523–530.

Lenneberg, E. (1967). 'Biological Foundations of Language'. John Wiley and Sons, New York.

Liberman, A. M., Cooper, F. S., Shankweiler, D. P. and Studdert-Kennedy, M. (1967). Perception of the speech code. *Psychol. Rev.* 74, 431–461.

Lowe, A. D. and Campbell, R. A. (1965). Temporal discrimination in aphasoid and normal children. *J. Speech. Hear. Res.* 8, 313–315.

Lowe, S., Berlin, C. I., Cullen, J. K. and Thompson, C. L. (1970). Dichotic simultaneous and time-staggered message perception in normals and patients with temporal lobe lesions. *Amer. Speech Hear. Assn.* (Abs.) 12, 423.

Lynn, G. E. and Gilroy, J. (1972). Neuro-audiological abnormalities in patients with temporal lobe tumors. *J. Neurol. Sci.* 17, 167–184.

Marin, O., Saffran, E. and Schwartz, M. F. (1976). Dissociations of language in aphasia: Implications for normal function. *Ann. N.Y. Acad. Sci.* 280, 864–884.

Mendel, M. I. (1974). Influence of stimulus level and sleep stage on the early components of the averaged electroencephalic response to clicks during all-night sleep. *J. Speech Hear. Res.* 17, 5–17.

Menyuk, P. (1964). A comparison of grammar of children with functionally deviant and normal speech. *J. Speech Hear. Res.* 7, 109–122.

Menyuk, P. (1974). The bases of language acquisition: Some questions. *J. Autism Child. Schizophr.* 4, 325–345.

Morehead, D. M. and Morehead, A. (1974). From Signal to Sign: A Piagetian View of Thought and Language During the First Two Years. *In* 'Language Perspectives – Acquisition, Retardation, and Intervention' (R. L. Schieffelbusch and L. L. Lloyd, eds), pp. 153–190. University Park Press, Baltimore, London and Tokyo.

Morley, M. E. (1972). 'The Development and Disorders of Speech in Childhood'. Churchill Livingstone, Edinburgh and London.

Peiper, A. (1963). 'Cerebral Function in Infancy and Childhood'. Consultants Bureau, New York.

Piaget, J. (1963). Le Langage et les Opérations Intellectuelles. *In* 'Problèmes de Psycholinguistique: Symposium de l'Association de Psychologie Scientifique de Langue Française'. Presses Universitaires de France, Paris.

Picton, T. W., Hillyard, S. A., Krautz, H. J. and Galambos, R. (1974). Human auditory evoked potentials I: Evaluation of components. *Electroenceph. clin. Neurophysiol.* 36, 179–190.

Poppen, R., Stark, J., Eisenson, J., Forrest, T. and Wertheim, G. (1969). Visual sequencing performance of aphasic children. *J. Speech Hear. Res.* **12**, 288–300.

Rapin, I. (1974). Testing for hearing loss with auditory evoked responses – successes and failures. *J. Commun. Dis.* **7**, 3–10.

Rapin, I. and Costa, L. D. (1969). Test-retest reliability of audiograms in children at a school for the deaf. *J. Speech Hear. Res.* **12**, 402–412.

Rapin, I., Mattis, S., Rowan, A. J. and Golden, G. G. (1977). Verbal auditory agnosia in children. *Develop. Med. Child Neurol.* **19**, 192–20.

Rapin, I. and Steinherz, P. (1970). Reaction time for pediatric audiometry. *J. Speech Hear. Res.* **13**, 203–217.

Rapin, I., Wilson, B. C., Wilson, J. J. and Allen, D. A. Neuropsychologic, neurologic and linguistic profiles in school age children with developmental language disabilities. Unpublished.

Rees, N. S. (1973). Auditory processing factors in language disorders: The view from Procrustes' bed. *J. Speech Hear. Dis.* **38**, 304–315.

Rutter, M. (ed.) (1971). 'Infantile Autism: Concepts, Characteristics and Treatment'. Churchill Livingstone, London.

Sachs, M. B. (ed.) (1971). 'Physiology of the Auditory System'. National Educational Consultants, Baltimore.

Schain, R. J. and Wiley, J. (1965). Evolution of a characteristic speech disorder in juvenile cerebral lipidosis. *Trans. Amer. Neurol. Assoc.* **90**, 290–291.

Shriner, T. H., Holloway, M. S. and Daniloff, R. G. (1969). The relationship between articulatory deficits and syntax in speech defective children. *J. Speech Hear. Res.* **12**, 319–325.

Simmons, F. B. and Russ, F. M. (1974). Automated newborn hearing screening, the Crib-o-gram. *Acta oto-lar.* **100**, 1–7.

Stein, L. K. and Curry, F. K. W. (1968). Childhood auditory agnosia. *J. Speech Hear. Dis.* **33**, 361–370.

Steinschneider, A., Lipton, E. L. and Richmond, J. B. (1966). Auditory sensitivity in the infant: Effect of intensity on cardiac and motor responsivity. *Child Devel.* **37**, 234–252.

Tallal, P. and Piercy, M. (1973a). Defects of non-verbal auditory perception in children with developmental aphasia. *Nature* **241**, 468–469.

Tallal, P. and Piercy, M. (1973b). Developmental aphasia: Impaired rate of non-verbal processing as a function of sensory modality. *Neuropsychologia* **11**, 389–398.

Wada, J. A., Clarke, R. and Hamm, A. (1975). Cerebral hemispheric asymmetry in humans. Cortical speech zones in 100 adult and 100 infant brains. *Arch. Neurol.* **32**, 239–246.

Warrington, E. K., Logue, V. and Pratt, R. T. C. (1971). The anatomical localization of selective impairment of auditory verbal short-term memory. *Neuropsychologia* **9**, 377–387.

Wedenberg, E. (1956). Auditory tests on newborn infants. *Acta oto-lar.* **46**, 446–461.

Wilber, L. A. (1974). Significance and detection of conductive lesions in children with multiple handicaps. *J. Commun. Dis.* **7**, 31–44.

Wilson, B. C., Wilson, J. J. and Allen, D. A. Neuropsychologic, neurologic and linguistic profiles in preschool age children with developmental language disabilities. Unpublished.

Witelson, S. F. and Pallie, W. (1973). Left hemisphere specialization for language in the newborn. Neuroanatomical evidence of asymmetry. *Brain* **96**, 641–646.

Worster-Drought, C. (1971). An unusual form of acquired aphasia in children. *Develop. Med. Child Neurol.* **13**, 563–571.

Yoss, K. A. and Darley, F. L. (1974). Developmental apraxia of speech in children with defective articulation. *J. Speech Hear. Res.* **17**, 399–416.

The Cognitive Functioning
of Children with
Developmental Dysphasia

Arthur Benton

Introduction

The status of cognitive processes in children with developmental dysphasia is of importance in two respects. From a theoretical standpoint, information about the level and pattern of intellectual functioning of these children is necessary for a satisfactory understanding of the nature of their rather puzzling disorders of speech and language. From a practical standpoint, the nurture and education of these children should be consonant with the level of their cognitive capacities.

It is generally recognised that developmental dysphasia is a collective term covering a variety of conditions involving failure or distortion in the development of speech and language. A division into two broad categories of disturbance, expressive and receptive-expressive, is widely accepted. The child with an expressive (or predominantly expressive) language disorder shows a level of understanding of oral speech that is significantly higher than his oral speech production. His understanding of oral speech may be mildly or moderately subnormal but the expressive speech disorder, which is his primary problem, is always more severe. In contrast, the central feature of the clinical picture presented by the child with receptive-expressive speech disorder is his disability in understanding oral speech. Distortion or impoverishment in speech expression is invariably a part of the syndrome but the receptive defect is considered to be primary.

A number of conditions may be distinguished within the category of developmental expressive dysphasia. One group of children is clearly dysarthric. These are children, many with frank cerebral palsy, whose primary problem is defective neuromotor control of the organs of speech articulation. Where neurological disorder is not clearly evident, the speech defect itself is sometimes interpreted as a sign of 'minimal' cerebral palsy and sometimes as an expression of delayed cerebral maturation. Unless there are complicating factors in addition to the neuromuscular disability, understanding of oral speech and silent reading are expected to be within the normal range.

A second group of children show less consistent disturbances in articulation. They may block and misarticulate in spontaneous and conversational speech but generally perform better in test situations involving the repetition of sounds or the naming of objects. Their disabilities do not appear to be a direct consequence of sensorimotor defects but rather of impairment of coordination or integration in the absence of paresis or ataxia. Again, significant defects in language understanding and reading are not viewed as essential parts of the clinical picture.

The expressive speech of a third group of children in this category is characterised more by lexical and syntactic impoverishment than by defective articulation, although the latter may be present. These 'quiet' children produce little spontaneous speech and give brief replies in conversation. When they talk, their speech is more or less telegraphic with frequent omission of conjunctions, prepositions and articles. They tend to speak in single words or short phrases rather than complete sentences. Use of gestures for the purpose of communication is variable. As these children mature, whatever articulatory defects they may have shown are likely to disappear but, although there is some improvement, the relative syntactic poverty of their expressive language persists and is manifested in writing as well as in oral speech. Language understanding and reading tend to be subnormal but only to a moderate degree.

Thus the first two groups of children in the 'expressive speech defect' category have a disability primarily affecting articulation and the programming of speech while the disability of the third group primarily involves the utilisation of language as a system. The first group corresponds to the 'motor' type and the second group to the 'language' type of developmental dysphasia described by Greene, 1960; Crookes and Greene, 1963. The feature that defines the category as a whole is the presence of a defect in expressive language with relatively intact language comprehension.

In contrast, as has been remarked, children with receptive-expressive dysphasia show serious impairment in the understanding of oral language. Moreover, their defects in expressive language are qualitatively of a different nature from those observed in the primarily expressive category. They may speak fluently but distort speech sounds, not because of articulatory difficulty, but seemingly because of defective self-monitoring mechanisms. These are the children to whom the labels, 'congenital word-deafness' and 'congenital auditory imperception' (Worster-Drought and Allen, 1929a, b) have been applied. The first term places emphasis on their verbal receptive disabilities as the core of the clinical picture and draws an analogy between the condition and acquired word deafness, as seen in adult patients. The second term implies a more comprehensive disorder in audioperceptual function extending beyond the understanding of linguistic material to encompass the discrimination and recognition of non-verbal sounds. The expressive speech characteristics of these children with receptive-expressive dysphasia vary from one case to another. Some say very little whilst others have evident articulatory difficulties. In the majority of cases, however, speech output is normal both in quantity and rate but is characterised by the occurrence of unintelligible neologisms so that the total effect is that of jargon speech or 'idioglossia' (Worster-Drought and Allen, 1930). A salient feature is the inability to imitate speech sounds, including those in the child's conversational repertory.

The diversity of conditions represented by the label, 'developmental aphasia', needs to be kept in mind when considering the status of cognitive abilities in these children. What may be true for one sub-group may not hold for another. Clinicians, such as Stambak (1959) and Crookes and Greene (1963), have described distinctive patterns of abilities and dis-abilities for different sub-groups. As will be seen, some studies deal with a mixture of sub-groups whilst others fail to describe adequately the defining characteristics of the investigated sample of children. No doubt this accounts in part for the large within-group variability reported in many studies.

Intelligence Level

By definition, the intelligence level of children with developmental aphasia, including those with severe receptive-expressive impairment, must be high enough to support the expectation either of adequate under-standing and expression of speech for age or of a level of language behaviour significantly higher than what is observed. When William Wilde (1853) first described children who were 'dumb but not deaf', he pointed out that some were neither 'paralytic nor idiotic'. If, according to the standards of the time, all these children had been judged to be 'idiots', Wilde would no doubt have viewed their impairment in expressive speech as simply a reflection of their pervasive mental retardation and would not have called specific attention to a sub-group that was not mentally defective.

It is customary to assess the intelligence level of language-handicapped children by means of standardised performance tests although, occasion-ally, a test battery consisting of both verbal and performance sub-tests has been employed for this purpose. Review of clinical and experimental studies in which these test batteries have been utilised indicates that there is great variation in intelligence in this clinical population. Many dysphasic children are demonstrably of high average or moderately superior intelligence. An unduly large number, however, seem to be low or dull average and there is a strong suggestion that, in addition to greater variability, a group trend towards a lower level of 'general intelligence' than would be expected, in the light of background factors, exists. The information provided in some recent studies will be considered from this standpoint.

Gordon and Taylor (1964), in their analysis of the problems associated with the clinical evaluation of children with language disorders, describe the characteristics of a sub-group of 12 cases (mostly of the receptive-expressive type) which they selected as representative of the total sample of children seen in their clinic. Eight children were judged to be intellectually subnormal (IQ < 90), two were judged to be average and two to be above average in intelligence. In contrast, the mean IQ of the 80 dysphasic children with either expressive or receptive-expressive impairment studied by Ingram (1959) was about 102, with 23 children showing Terman-Merrill IQs of 110 or higher as compared to 15 children with IQs of 89 or lower. The socio-economic background of the group was, however, quite atypical. About 46 per cent of the children came from the two highest social classes (defined by parental occupation) whereas, in the Scottish population an estimated 12·5 per cent of dysphasic children belong to these classes. Conversely, 7·5 per cent came from the lowest social class as compared to an estimated frequency of about 14·5 per cent in this class in the population. In view of this bias, the observed mean IQ of the clinical group may have been somewhat below expectations. But the employment of an intelligence scale with verbal sub-tests, such as the Terman-Merrill, makes interpretation difficult.

Experimental studies designed to investigate specific cognitive functions in language-handicapped children generally exclude those with clearly subnormal intelligence in order to permit an unequivocal interpretation of the meaning of the task performances. Thus the study of Weiner (1969) of perceptual performances in children with expressive language disorders involved a sample of eight children with a mean non-verbal IQ (Arthur Adaptation of the Leiter International Performance Scale) of 103 (SD = 10·6) with a range of 88–118. The children of the control group with whom the language-handicapped children were individually matched had a mean IQ of 99 (SD = 7·5) with a range of 91–109 and, as a group, were slightly lower in respect to socio-economic status. The greater variability of the clinical sample, despite the attempt to match pairs of subjects on an individual basis, is evident. Tallal and Piercy (1973a, b), in their studies of auditory information processing in dysphasic children (most of them of the receptive-expressive type), dealt with a sample of 12 children with a mean performance test IQ of 108, the range being 85–127. In the absence of information about selection procedures and the socioeconomic background of the experimental and the control group (whose IQ scores are not reported), it is not possible to infer whether or not the mean IQ score of 108 conforms to expectations. But one cannot but be impressed by the wide variation in scores in this very small group.

Stark (1967) selected 30 dysphasic children for study on the basis 'of a disparity between non-verbal and verbal ability'. Their mean IQ score on the Arthur Adaptation of the Leiter International Performance Scale was 96 (SD = 13) as compared to a mean Stanford-Binet IQ of 77 (SD = 14). Thus, despite the selective bias, the non-verbal intelligence of the sample proved to be rather low. A comparative study by Black (1973) of the performances of dysphasic children on the Arthur Adaptation of the Leiter International Performance Scale and Peabody Picture Vocabulary Test also provides data suggesting somewhat depressed non-verbal intelligence in these children. The mean Leiter IQ of this sample of 100 children (almost all of whom were developmental dysphasics) was 82 (SD = 18) while the mean Picture Vocabulary IQ was 69 (SD = 17).

Thus the weight of evidence suggests that dysphasic children show greater than normal variability in 'general intelligence' as well as a group trend towards a lower than expected IQ. Two possible reasons for these findings will be considered.

CONCURRENCE OF DEVELOPMENTAL DYSPHASIA AND MENTAL SUBNORMALITY

One possibility is that the variability in intelligence level is related to a corresponding variability in the cerebral abnormality underlying the specific language disability. In the case of some children, the cerebral abnormality may be limited in extent and thus affect only those functions involved in speech and language learning. In the case of other children, the cerebral abnormality may be sufficiently extensive to retard their general intellectual development as well as have a specific effect on the acquisition of language skills. The fact that frank mental retardation is often associated with striking abnormalities of speech and language is consistent with the latter possibility. For example, many researchers have noted an excessively high frequency of defects in speech articulation among the mentally retarded as compared to younger normal children of the same mental age (Benton, 1964a). The significance of brain disease as a determinant of speech defect is reflected in the observation that retardates in the 'brain-damaged' categories generally show a higher frequency of articulation defects than do those in the 'cultural-familial' or 'subcultural' category (Schlanger and Gottesleben, 1957; Blanchard, 1964). There is also evidence that many retardates show pronounced impairment in the development of linguistic functions that cannot be accounted for by their low mental age (Lyle, 1961; Lovell and Bradbury, 1967).

Thus a possible explanation for the greater variability in intelligence (determined for the most part by the more frequent occurrence of subnormal cases) among dysphasic children is what may be called the 'concurrence hypothesis'. As indicated, it ascribes the observed association to the variable effects of brain disease on both intellectual and linguistic functions. The hypothesis denies an integral relationship between the language disability and intelligence level.

LANGUAGE DISABILITY AS A DEPRIVATION FACTOR

Another possibility which deserves to be considered is that the child's dysphasia restricts (or distorts) his life experiences seriously enough to cause a general retardation in his intellectual growth. On this view, specific language disability may be expected to operate like any other handicapping factor, such as physical impairment, cultural impoverishment or even emotional disturbance, to diminish a child's opportunities for learning intellectual skills. That there is an overall negative association between these disabilities and intelligence level is undeniable. For example, surveys of the distribution of intelligence in the blind and the deaf generally indicate a mean IQ which is about 10 points below normative standards (Hayes, 1941, 1950; Wiley, 1971). The measured intelligence and social competence of many of these handicapped children are low enough to lead to their classification as mentally retarded.

Yet, given the observed association between these disabilities and subnormal intelligence, the extent to which they function to depress intellectual growth is uncertain. For example, in the case of physically or culturally handicapped retardates, the problem of distinguishing those who are 'truly' retarded *and* have a specific handicap from those who are retarded *by reason of* the handicap (i.e. who are 'pseudo-retarded') is one of long standing and is still far from being resolved (Arthur, 1947; Delay *et al.*, 1952; Benton, 1956, 1964a, 1970; Dawson *et al.*, 1956; Bialer, 1970). The tremendous variability in intelligence among the physically handicapped and the systematic relationship of intelligence level to specific clinical types of disability also cast doubt about the importance of the handicap itself as a depressing agent. Thus the observation that blind children 'as a group' score about 10 points below normative expectations is not very meaningful in the light of the wide disparity among sub-groups within the category. A majority of children with congenital anophthalmos show frank mental retardation (Bachelis, 1967). In contrast, those who are blind as a consequence of retinoblastoma are generally of superior intelligence (Thurrell and Josephson, 1966; Williams, 1968). In both conditions, the blindness *per se* can play only a minor role, if any, in determining the rate and limits of intellectual growth.

These reservations do not rule out the possibility that there are situations in which a sensory or motor handicap does exert a significant, if not an overriding, influence on intellectual development, particularly if the handicap exists in combination with other adverse factors. Clinicians and teachers rather expect that a neglected blind child or a child whose deafness has gone unrecognised will show subnormal intelligence. In instances such as these it is reasonable to conceive of the intellectual retardation as the consequence of the interaction between the sensory or motor handicap and the environmental mishandling (see Benton, 1970, for illustrative case histories and a model depicting intelligence level as the resultant of multiple interacting determinants). Thus, although clear evidence is lacking, specific sensory, motor or emotional disability cannot be dismissed as a possible determinant of general intellectual level.

It is possible to view developmental dysphasia, particularly of the receptive-expressive type, as another such specific handicapping factor because, in the absence of special environmental measures, it must surely operate to restrict the range and variety of a child's experiences as well as his capacity to engage in meaningful transactions with other people. An incidental observation by Landau *et al.* (1960) in their study of a child with receptive-expressive dysphasia may be cited to illustrate the point. When first seen, this six-year-old boy had practically no understanding of oral language and spoke an incomprehensibe jargon. His IQ score on a performance test battery was 78. Over the course of the next three years, he was given intensive language training and made considerable progress. He could produce simple sentences that were grammatically correct, had a fair vocabulary and developed some understanding of oral speech. Retested at the age of nine years, his 'non-verbal' IQ was found to be 97. The mechanisms involved in this remarkable rise in 'non-verbal' IQ in conjunction with improvement in language skills are, of course, unknown. That the boy's steadily increasing linguistic efficiency permitted him to engage in learning experiences which accelerated his general mental development is surely a tenable hypothesis.

Specific Cognitive Disabilities and Developmental Dysphasia

Proceeding from the premise that the possession of one or another specific cognitive capacity is a prerequisite for the normal growth of speech and language, a number of hypotheses have attempted to relate developmental dysphasia to impairment in these capacities. On this view, the dysphasia is not an independent disorder but a particular expression of a more basic cognitive impairment influencing non-verbal as well as verbal behaviour. As Affolter *et al.* (1974b) have phrased it: disturbances of language are secondary to disturbances of perception of a pre-verbal nature.

One such hypothesis ascribes developmental dysphasia of the receptive-expressive type to higher-level audioperceptual impairment (Worster-Drought and Allen, 1929a, b, 1930; Benton, 1964b; Tallal and Piercy, 1973a, b, 1974, 1975). 'Higher-level' impairment is intended here to mean defective processing of auditory information within the context of adequate reception of the information, in contrast to deafness which implies inadequate reception. The distorted development of receptive and expressive language in the dysphasic child is seen as a direct result of his inability to discriminate and identify complex auditory stimuli, which include, but are not limited to, speech sounds. Since this topic is treated in detail in the chapter by Tallal and Piercy on defects in auditory perception, it will be considered here only when the question of modality-specific versus more general defect is raised. Other types of cognitive deficit that have been proposed as the *Grundstörung* underlying developmental dysphasia are of a 'supramodal' nature, i.e. not specifically associated with a single sensory modality.

DEFECTS IN SEQUENTIAL PERCEPTION

The leading hypothesis of this kind is that the capacity to integrate successively presented stimuli into a unitary perception or, on the motor side, to organise movements into an integrated temporal pattern is essential for language acquisition and that, at least in some children, developmental dysphasia can be ascribed to defect in this capacity. This theoretical position was stated in general terms by Lashley (1951) who pointed out that conventional language usage in both its expressive and receptive aspects necessarily implies the existence of schemata or dispositions which permit the orderly temporal integration of the elements of speech. Similarly, Efron (1963) postulated that correct appreciation of the temporal order of stimulation is essential to the processing and production of speech. The implications of this hypothesis have been investigated in a number of studies of the perception of temporal order in adult patients with acquired aphasia as compared to brain-diseased patients without aphasia and normal controls (cf. Efron, 1963; Edwards and Auger, 1965; Holmes, 1965; Brookshire, 1972; Swisher and Hirsh, 1972). The results suggest that aphasic patients are impaired in the perception of the temporal order of *auditory* stimuli, non-verbal as well as verbal. In contrast, the performances of aphasics on tasks requiring discrimination of the temporal order of visual stimuli appear to be comparable to those of non-aphasics. This pattern of findings has been interpreted by Swisher and Hirsh (1972) to mean that, whilst a central neural system for temporal ordering, independent of sensory modality, may exist, impaired functioning of such a system cannot be invoked as the basis for aphasic disorder.

Application of this concept to the problem of developmental dysphasia was suggested by Monsees (1961) who expressed the belief 'that the core of the language disability is a disorder in the perception of temporal sequence, auditory and perhaps visual'. The hypothesis has been put to test in a number of studies.

Furth (1964) investigated visual sequence learning in dysphasic, deaf and normal children. Ten children, diagnosed as 'sensory aphasic', who showed severe disturbances in both receptive and expressive language, constituted the experimental group. The children ranged in age from 9 to 14 years (mean = 10·6 years). Their mean WISC Performance Scale IQ was 101. An incidental, and possibly relevant, finding was that the children's lowest scores were on Picture Arrangement, a test requiring temporospatial ordering of information. The deaf control group consisted of 10 children who were matched with the aphasics on the basis of performance on a 'discrete' paired-associate learning task, as described below. The normal control group consisted of 10 children who were matched with the dysphasics for sex, IQ and performance on the 'discrete' paired-associate learning task. Both the normal and deaf groups consisted of children in the 10–11 years age range.

Meaningless figures, taken from the list of Vanderplas and Garvin (1959), were utilised as stimuli in the learning tasks. In the 'discrete' task, the subjects were required to learn responses to single figures. As mentioned, the three groups were matched for performance level on this task. In the 'simultaneous sequence' task, the subjects learned responses to sequences of two figures presented simultaneously. In the 'successive sequence' task, they learned responses to two figures presented in succession. The deaf and normal children did not differ in performance on either of the sequential tasks. The dysphasic children performed on a lower level than either control group on each sequential task. None of the between-groups differences, however, was statistically significant. Thus, although the findings were in the direction predicted by the hypothesis, they did not offer strong support for it. Both the small size of the contrasting groups and the high within-group variability, however, militated against finding significant differences between them. Inspection of the ranges of scores suggests that the three groups were about equally variable on the discrete and simultaneous sequence tasks but that the dysphasic children showed greater variability than the controls on the successive sequence task. Assuming this to be the case, it is quite possible that analysis of individual performances would have brought to light a sub-group of dysphasic children who performed on a 'pathologically' low level on the successive sequence task, as defined by scores below the distributions of the control groups.

In a second study, Furth and Pufall (1965) presented tasks of a similar nature to groups of hearing-impaired children who differed in respect to their rate of progress in language learning under conventional teaching conditions. Those who had made poor progress and had been assigned to a special teaching division were classified as 'aphasic'. No significant between-groups differences were found for any of the visual learning tasks, sequential or non-sequential. The younger 'aphasic' children (6–7 years) were decidedly inferior to the controls on an auditory sequencing task but the older groups (10–11 years) did not differ in performance level. Both hearing-impaired groups performed more poorly than did normal hearing children of comparable intelligence level.

Lowe and Campbell (1965) compared small groups of normal and 'aphasoid' children (some of whom 'had possible minimal hearing losses') on tasks requiring the auditory discrimination of succession or temporal order. Two 1000 Hz tones were the stimuli in the succession task in which the children had to report whether they heard 1 or 2 tones. The mean temporal interval at which the tones could be discriminated as occurring in succession was 18·5 ms for the normal children and 35·8 ms for the 'aphasoids', the between-groups difference was not significant. Judging from the reported ranges of scores, the 'aphasoid' children were more variable than the controls. A 2200 Hz and a 400 Hz tone were employed in the temporal order task. Here the mean intervals at which order of the two tones could be correctly identified were 36·1 ms for the normal children and 257·0 ms for the 'aphasoids', the large between-groups difference being significant at the 0·005 level. The authors conclude that impaired perception of temporal order is a significant feature of childhood dysphasia and may be an important determinant of these children's problem in communication.

This study was the subject of a critique by Campanelli (1966) who pointed out that it suffered from a number of defects which made a meaningful interpretation of the findings difficult. The bases for the classification of the children as 'aphasoid' are not specified. The statement that some children suffered from 'possible minimal hearing loss' is too indefinite to be informative. If such loss involved the higher frequencies, it is possible that perception of the 2200 Hz tone in the temporal order task was impaired to a sufficient degree to affect performance on that task. In a subsequent note, Campbell (1967) stated that some of the 8 children showed pure-tone thresholds indicative of mild to moderate losses in the 500–2000 Hz range.

Stark (1967) compared the performances of 30 dysphasic children (mean age, 6 years, 6 months) on three sequencing tests with normative standards derived from their standardisation. The tests were the Auditory-Vocal Sequencing and Visual-Motor Sequencing sub-tests of the Illinois Test of Psycholinguistic Abilities (Kirk and McCarthy, 1961) and the Knox Cubes test (cf. Corkin, 1974). The children scored below the standardisation means on all three tests, the discrepancy between observed and expected performance being much larger for the auditory tasks than for either visual task. While performances on the two visual tests were positively correlated to a moderate degree (r = 0·41), neither test showed a correlation with auditory test performance. As noted earlier, the mean Leiter IQ of this sample of children was 96. Thus the outcome of the study suggested a significant defect in auditory sequencing but only a mild impairment in visual sequencing.

Evidence for mildly defective visual sequencing capacity in dysphasic children was also adduced in a series of studies by Poppen et al. (1969). The subjects were children with both receptive and expressive defects whose non-verbal intelligence was within the average range. Hearing loss, although present in some cases, could not be made to account for the language disability. On tasks involving the reproduction of sequences of lights, the mean error rates of the dysphasics were significantly higher than those of age-matched normal children. The performance level of the dysphasic children on these visual tasks was, however, considerably better than that found for a comparable auditory task in an earlier study (Stark et al., 1967).

Tallal and Piercy (1973a, b, 1974, 1975), whose studies have demonstrated the critical importance of the variables of stimulus duration and interstimulus interval as determinants of the accuracy of auditory perception in children with receptive-expressive dysphasic disorder, found that these children performed normally on tasks requiring the visual discrimination of temporal order. In contrast, they were notably deficient in performance on comparable tasks in the auditory modality.

Most recently, Kracke (1975) has reported a study of the perception of rhythmic sequences by dysphasic, deaf and normal children in which striking differences between the aphasics and the control groups were found. Twelve aphasic children of the receptive-expressive type were matched with deaf and normal children for non-verbal intelligence, age and sex. The children ranged in age from 8 to 15 years and in no case was the intelligence level less than low average (WISC performance Scale IQ above 90). The stimulus sequences were simple rhythmic patterns presented in either the auditory or the tactile modality. These were presented in pairs, the child being required to judge whether the members of the pair were the same or different. The deaf and the normal children found both tasks fairly easy, the percentage of correct responses being 86 per cent (deaf) and 97 per cent (normal) for the auditory modality and 92 per cent (deaf) and 88 per cent (normal) for the tactile modality. The dysphasic children showed an impaired performance on both tasks, the percentage of correct responses being 55 per cent for the auditory modality and 49 per cent for the tactile modality. Variability was great with some children performing above and some definitely below the level of chance success. Since the dysphasic children's performance on the tactile task was as poor as on the auditory task, Kracke concludes that their disability in the recognition of rhythmic sequences is of a supramodal nature.

OTHER COGNITIVE DEFECTS

As the preceding section indicates, a substantial amount of empirical study has been devoted to the question of whether dysphasic children show a specific deficit in the apprehension of temporal sequences, as measured by tasks requiring the discrimination of succession, temporal order and rhythmic patterns. Other aspects of non-verbal cognition, which from time to time have been suggested as related to their linguistic disability, have been the subject of only a few scattered studies.

Since impairment in higher-level visuoperceptive functions has been so often implicated as a salient disability in children with brain damage, 'minimal brain dysfunction' and 'learning disabilities', it is natural that these functions should have been invesigated in dysphasic children; the working hypothesis being that the adequate development of these ca- pacities is one of the 'pre-verbal' prerequisites for normal speech and language development (cf. Affolter et al., 1974a, b). For the most part, the available empirical findings do not confirm this hypothesis. In the study by Crookes and Greene (1963) of children with 'motor' and 'lan- guage' types of dysphasia, the Block Designs sub-test of the WISC was among those given to the children. In both groups, performance on the test was somewhat higher than their IQ scores. The 'motor' group ob- tained a mean scale score of 13·3 on Block Designs, as compared to their mean IQ of 114; the mean scale score of the 'language' group was 10·6, as compared to their mean IQ of 101. The dysphasic children in the study of Furth (1964) also performed on an average level on the WISC Block Designs, which was consonant with their performance scale IQ of 101. Similarly, Weiner (1969) found that the Bender-Gestalt and 'Draw-A- Person' test performances of his dysphasic children were not poorer than those of their matched controls.

A study that did, in fact, adduce evidence for inferior visuospatial func- tioning in dysphasic children of the receptive-expressive type is that of Doehring (1960) who assessed memory for the location of visual stimuli in normal, deaf and dysphasic school age subjects. The normal and deaf groups performed at about the same level and both were significantly superior to the aphasic group. As Doehring points out, however, the mean non-verbal IQ of the dysphasics was about 10 points lower than those of the control groups and, at the same time, accuracy of visual localisation was correlated to a modest degree (r = 0·25–0·33) with IQ. Thus it can be assumed that the differences in task performance would have been somewhat less in groups equated for IQ.

Audiovisual associative learning in receptive-expressive aphasic children and a mixed group of deaf and hearing children was studied by Wilson et al. (1960). The experimental task consisted of the presentation of different paired sounds and visually displayed letters of the alphabet. As a group, the dysphasic children performed at a lower level than the controls but the more striking finding was the wide range of scores in the dysphasic group. All 13 children in the control group achieved the criterion of learning within 50 trials while 6 of the 14 dysphasic children failed to reach criterion in 80 trials. On the other hand, the 3 fastest learners in the dysphasic group reached criterion in almost as few trials as the 3 fastest controls. The other 5 dysphasic children reached criterion in less than 65 trials. The authors suggest further exploration of the hypothesis that a specific disability in learning intermodal associations is characteristic of a sub-group of dysphasic children.

Mackworth et al. (1973) have reported differences in the orienting response of normal and dysphasic children to the appearance of a new visual stimulus. The children were instructed to look at a repetitively presented display of white geometric shapes. After 10 presentations, the colour of one of the 16 shapes was changed to red and the new display repetitively presented. The orienting response and subsequent habituation were assessed by recording the direction of gaze. While the normal children showed the orienting response followed by habituation, reflected by a progressive decrease in the amount of time spent in gazing at the red figure, the dysphasics (most of whom were of the receptive-expressive type) showed much less habituation. Those classified as most severely dysphasic showed virtually no adaptation. The authors offer the interpretation that this failure in adaptation results from a selective defect in forming an internal neural model of the environment, the latter being a necessary precondition for the extinction of an orienting response.

Concluding Comments

This review of the literature on cognitive functions in children with developmental dysphasia has not been exhaustive. Many contributions have not been mentioned, primarily because of their failure to provide essential background information or because defects in their design render the reported findings uninterpretable. The one area which has been considered in some detail is that of sequential perception, since so much attention has been focused on the question of whether dysphasic children show specific impairment in this area.

Several studies have investigated different aspects of verbal performance in dysphasic children with the aim of identifying the cognitive deficits that may underlie their speech and language problems. Audio-vocal repetition (of vowels, nonsense syllables, words and sentences) and grasp of syntactic constructions are among the performances that have been most frequently assessed and impairment on the part of dysphasic children has been a virtually constant finding (cf. Ajuriaguerra et al., 1965; Weiner, 1969) From such observations it is sometimes inferred that these children, or at least a sub-group of them, are defective in 'gestalt formation' or in the ordering of experience in time and space with the implication that the deficiency is responsible for the failure in speech and language development.

These findings, and the supportive observations of clinicians, are valuable on a descriptive level and they provide useful guides for the special education of dysphasic children. They are equally valuable as a source of research hypotheses. But the validation of these hypotheses, which implicate cognitive deficits of a basic nature as determinants of developmental dysphasia, requires that these cognitive functions be studied in connection with appropriate tasks that do not involve the very modes of reception and expression in which the child is deficient. The experimental task must be of a non-verbal nature or, if a linguistic hypothesis is being tested, it must involve modes of reception (e.g. vision) and response (e.g. gesture or pantomime) other than those which are the core characteristics of the dysphasic disability.

As has been noted, there is a trend in dysphasic children towards a somewhat lower than expected level of general intelligence, as assessed by non-verbal tests, in dysphasic children. In view of a bias towards the exclusion of mentally retarded subjects in the identification, study and treatment of dysphasic children, this observation probably represents a real phenomenon. Possible determinants of the trend have been considered. In some cases, the underlying cerebral abnormality may produce both a dysphasic disorder and some degree of general mental subnormality. In other cases, the dysphasia itself may be responsible for a condition of experiential deprivation that retards general mental development. Receptive-expressive disability should be more potent than predominantly expressive disability in this regard and there is a suggestion that this is the case, i.e. that receptive-expressive aphasics show mental subnormality more frequently than do expressive aphasics. This 'cultural deprivation' hypothesis is important from a practical standpoint for it clearly implies that appropriate environmental modifications designed to permit dysphasic children to expand the range of their experiences and activities should prevent or eliminate the general intellectual retardation that many of them show.

The considerable amount of research done on sequential perception and learning in dysphasic children bears witness to the importance which clinicians and investigators ascribe to defect in this cognitive capacity as a component of the language disorder. Specific training in sequential activities is a prominent feature of educational programmes for these children (cf. Barry, 1961; McGinnis, 1963). The empirical findings indicate clearly that significant defect in the apprehension of *auditory* temporal sequences is characteristic of many dysphasic children (Lowe and Campbell, 1965; Stark *et. al.*, 1967; Tallal and Piercy, 1973a; Kracke, 1975). It is not clear, however, that the impairment extends beyond the auditory modality. Studies of visual sequencing performance have yielded evidence of either a rather mild defect (Furth, 1964; Stark, 1967; Poppen *et al.*, 1969) or of no defect at all (Furth and Pufall, 1965; Tallal and Piercy, 1973b). The independence of auditory and visual sequencing capacity is suggested not only by the observed instances of dissociation in performance level but also by the lack of correlation between auditory and visual test performances found by Stark (1967). Kracke (1975), however, did find comparable impairment in the tactile and auditory perception of rhythmic patterns in children with receptive-expressive dysphasia. Further study along this line needs to be undertaken. Confirmation of this finding would be most interesting in view of the close connection between the two sensory modalities.

In summary, evidence to date indicates that failure in sequential tasks does not represent a cognitive defect which is independent of sensory modality but rather one which is specifically associated with audition. As has been noted, the same pattern of results has been found in adult patients with acquired aphasia who show impaired auditory, but intact visual, perception of temporal order. The most reasonable interpretation of these findings would seem to point to a distinctive defect in the auditory perception of children with receptive-expressive dysphasia (cf. Tallal and Piercy, this volume).

Studies assessing visuoanalytic capacity and visual memory in dysphasic children have not yielded impressive findings. It does not seem that deficiencies in the visuoperceptual area can provide a useful explanation any more than they can with respect to developmental dyslexia.

Many studies have been directed to the question of the status of abstract reasoning and symbolic thinking in deaf children and adults and this, in fact, is one of the major issues in the field (cf. Furth, 1966). The same issue has always been a topic of major interest in the field of adult aphasia (Bay, 1962; Zangwill, 1964; De Renzi *et al.*, 1966; Archibald *et al.*, 1967). The role of impairment of symbolic processes in developmental dysphasia has been discussed by a number of authors (e.g. Kendall, 1966; Myklebust, 1971; Eisenson, 1971) and a distinction between the symbolic and non-symbolic components in the clinical picture is sometimes made. Ajuria-guerra *et al.* (1965) have reported a number of observations on reasoning and symbolic behaviour, as assessed by the Piaget-Inhelder tests, in a few dysphasic children of the predominantly expressive type. Their descriptions suggest a deficit in abstract reasoning on these tests which are largely of a verbal nature.

Systematic controlled studies of conceptual thinking, as assessed by appropriate non-verbal tests, have yet to be done. The Leiter International Performance Scale includes a variety of tasks assessing perceptual discrimination, constructional ability and conceptual thinking. Analysis of the test profiles of dysphasic children, with special reference to level of performance on the conceptual as compared to the non-conceptual tests, should prove informative. Other non-verbal tests of abstract reasoning that have been utilised with deaf and aphasic subjects may also be applied to dysphasic children. Given the close relationship between abstract thought and language function, the study of conceptual and symbolic thinking in dysphasic children would seem to offer a particularly fruitful line of inquiry. The identification of a sub-group of developmental dysphasics with specific impairment in abstract thinking would not only be of theoretical interest but also of considerable practical importance in indicating the directions which the special education of these children should take.

A closely related question that deserves serious attention concerns the ability of dysphasic children to utilise gesture and pantomime for purposes of communication. In the field of adult aphasia, the 'language of gesture' has been viewed as a means of assessing the degree to which aphasic disorder represents an impairment in symbolisation transcending conventional oral and written language. Case studies of dysphasic children sometimes include descriptions of their gestural behaviour. They appear to show great variability in this regard. Some make liberal use of gestures and pantomime in their attempts to communicate while others never resort to these forms of symbolic-expressive behaviour. But neither the expressive nor the receptive aspect of gestural capacity in dysphasic children has been systematically investigated.

The test battery of Goodglass and Kaplan (1963) assessing pantomimic expression and that of Duffy *et al.* (1975) assessing the recognition of pantomime have been used successfully with adult aphasics. These batteries provide a substantial number of items from which a selection could be made to devise tests that would be appropriate for the evaluation of the understanding and expression of pantomime in children. The findings of studies along this line should indicate whether a general impairment in symbolic understanding and expression is an important component of developmental dysphasia. A possible outcome might be the isolation of a category 'asymbolic' dysphasic children from other categories whose language disorders result from other factors. If this should prove to be the case, an important advance in our understanding of childhood dysphasia will have been achieved.

The strategy of future research on cognitive functions in dysphasic children may be considered. As this review indicates, most of the studies in the area have been concerned with the status of a single cognitive ability such as sequential perception, perceptuomotor skill or associative learning. They have yielded useful findings, even if the specific questions posed have not always been conclusively answered.

But, by its very nature, this specific approach cannot provide a picture of the constellation of abilities and disabilities that may be characteristic of different types of childhood dysphasia. More comprehensive studies assessing diverse facets of cognitive functioning are required to achieve this goal. A few such studies have been attempted but their design and execution have been faulty and hence the reported findings are more provocative than informative. A comprehensive study of this type requires a large sample of carefully classified subjects, possibly a larger sample than is available at any single centre. A soundly designed collaborative project, involving the participation of a number of centres, offers the promise of providing the empirical data essential for a clearer understanding of the cognitive functions of dysphasic children.

References

Affolter, F., Brubaker, R. and Bischofsberger, W. (1974). Comparative studies between normal and language-disturbed children based on performance profiles. *Acta oto-lar.*, Suppl. **323**, 5–32.

Affolter, F. D., Brubaker, R. S., Stockman, I. J., Coastam, A. and Bischofsberger, W. (1974b). Prerequisites for speech development: visual, auditory and tactile pattern discrimination. *Med. Prog. Technol.* **2**, 93–102.

Ajuriaguerra, J. de, Jaeggi, A., Guiguard, F., Kocher, F., Maquard, M., Roth, S. and Schmid, E. (1965). Évolution et pronostic de la dysphasie chez l'enfant. *Psychiatrie de l'Enfant* **8**, 391–452.

Archibald, Y. M., Wepman, J. M. and Jones, L. V. (1967). Non-verbal cognitive performance in aphasic and nonaphasic brain damaged patients. *Cortex* **3**, 275–294.

Arthur, G. (1947). Pseudo-feeblemindness. *Amer. J. ment. Defic.* **52**, 137–142.

Bachelis, L. A. (1967). Developmental patterns of individuals with bilateral congenital anophthalmos. *New Outlook Blind* **61**, 113–119.
Barry, H. (1961). 'The Young Aphasic Child: Evaluation and Training'. Alexander Graham Bell Assoc., Washington, D.C.
Bay, E. (1962). Aphasia and non-verbal disorders of language. *Brain* **85**, 411–426.
Benton, A. L. (1956). The concept of pseudofeeblemindness. *Arch. Neurol. Psychiat.* **75**, 379–388.
Benton, A. L. (1964a). Psychological Evaluation and Differential Diagnosis. In 'Mental Retardation' (H. A. Stevens and R. Heber, eds), pp. 16–56. University of Chicago Press, Chicago and London.
Benton, A. L. (1964b). Developmental aphasia and brain damage. *Cortex* **1**, 40–52.
Benton, A. L. (1970). Interactive determinants of mental deficiency. In 'Social-Cultural Aspects of Mental Retardation' (H. C. Haywood, ed.), pp. 661–671. Appleton-Century-Crofts, New York.
Bialer, I. (1970). Relationship of Mental Retardation to Emotional Disturbance and Physical Disability. In 'Social-Cultural Aspects of Mental Retardation' (H. C. Haywood, ed.) pp 607–660. Appleton-Century-Crofts, New York.
Black, F. W. (1973). Use of the Leiter International Performance Scale with aphasic children. *J. Speech Hear. Res.* **16**, 530–533.
Blanchard, I. (1964). Speech pattern and etiology in mental retardation. *Amer. J. ment. Defic.* **68**, 612–617.
Brookshire, R. H. (1972). Visual and auditory sequencing by aphasic subjects. *J. Comm. Dis.* **5**, 259–269.
Campanelli, P. A. (1966). Comments on the research report of Lowe and Campbell. *J. Speech Hear. Res.* **9**, 318.
Campbell, R. A. (1967). Re: Campanelli re: Lowe and Campbell's research report. *J. Speech Hear. Res.* **10**, 153–154.
Corkin, S. (1974). Serial-ordering deficits in inferior readers. *Neuropsychologia* **12**, 347–354.
Crookes, T. G. and Greene, M. C. L. (1963). Some characteristics of children with two types of speech disorders. *Brit. J. educ. Psychol.* **33**, 31–40.
Dawson, M. E., Evans, M. J., Reed, M. and Minski, L. (1956). An investigation into children in attempt to differentiate between mental defect and deafness. *J. ment. Sci.* **102**, 121–128.
Delay, J., Pichot, P. and Perse, J. (1952). La notion de débilité mentale camouflée. *Ann. Medico-psychol.* **110**, 615–619.
De Renzi, E., Faglioni, P., Savoiardo, M. and Vignolo, L. A. (1966). The influence of aphasia and of the hemispheric side of the cerebral lesion on abstract thinking. *Cortex* **2**, 399–420.
Doehring, D. G. (1960). Visual-spatial memory in aphasic children. *J. Speech Hear. Res.* **3**, 138–149.
Duffy, R. J., Duffy, J. R. and Pearson, K. L. (1975). Pantomime recognition in aphasics. *J. Speech Hear. Res.* **18**, 115–132.
Edwards, A. E. and Auger, R. (1965). 'The Effect of Aphasia on the Perception of Precedence'. Proc. 73rd Amer. Psychol. Assn. Convention, 207–208.
Efron, R. (1963). Temporal perception, aphasia, and déjà-vu. *Brain* **86**, 403–424.
Eisenson, J. (1971). Aphasia in Adults. In 'Handbook of Speech Pathology and

Audiology' (L. E. Travis, ed.), pp. 1219–1252. Appleton-Century-Crofts, New York.

Furth, H. G. (1964). Sequence learning in aphasic and deaf children. *J. Speech Hear. Dis.* **29**, 171–177.

Furth, H. G. (1966). 'Thinking Without Language'. Free Press, New York.

Furth, H. G. and Pufall, P. B. (1965). Visual and auditory sequence learning in hearing-impaired children. *J. Speech Hear. Res.* **9**, 441–449.

Goodglass, H. and Kaplan, E. (1963). Disturbances of gesture and pantomine in aphasia. *Brain* **86**, 703–720.

Gordon, N. and Taylor, I. G. (1964). The assessment of children with difficulties of communication. *Brain* **87**, 121–140.

Greene, M. C. L. (1960). Diagnosis and treatment of late speech and language development in children. *Folia Phoniat.* **12**, 101–107.

Hayes, S. P. (1941). 'Contributions to a Psychology of Blindness'. American Foundation for the Blind, New York.

Hayes, S. P. (1950). Measuring the Intelligence of the Blind. *In* 'Blindness' (P. A. Zahl, ed.), pp. 141–173. Princeton University Press, Princeton.

Holmes, H. (1965). Disordered perception of auditory sequential patterns in aphasia. Ph.D. Thesis, Harvard University.

Ingram, T. T. S. (1959). Specific developmental disorders of speech in childhood. *Brain* **82**, 450–467.

Kendall, D. C. (1966). Language and Communication Problems in Children. *In* 'Speech Pathology' (R. W. Rieber and R. S. Brubaker, eds), pp. 285–298. North-Holland Publishing Co., Amsterdam.

Kirk, S. A. and McCarthy, J. J. (1961). The Illinois test of linguistic abilities – an approach to differential diagnosis. *Amer. J. ment. Defic.* **66**, 399–412.

Kracke, I. (1975). Perception of rhythmic sequences by receptive aphasic and deaf children. *Brit. J. Dis. Comm.* **10**, 43–51.

Landau, W. M., Goldstein, R. and Kleffner, F. R. (1960). Congenital aphasia. A clinicopathologic study. *Neurology* 10, 915–921.

Lashley, K. S. (1951). The Problem of Serial Order in Behavior. *In* 'Cerebral Mechanisms in Behavior' (L. A. Jeffress, ed.), pp. 112–136. Wiley, New York.

Lovell, K. and Bradbury, B. (1967). The learning of English morphology in educationally subnormal special school children. *Amer. J. ment. Defic.* **71**, 609–615.

Lowe, A. D. and Campbell, R. A. (1965). Temporal discrimination in aphasoid and normal children. *J. Speech Hear. Res.* **8**, 313–314.

Lyle, J. G. (1961). Comparison of the language of normal and imbecile children. *J. ment. Defic. Res.* **5**, 40–51.

Mackworth, N. H., Grandstaff, N. W. and Pribram, K. H. (1973). Orientation to pictorial novelty by speech-disordered children. *Neuropsychologia* **11**, 443–450.

McGinnis, M. (1963). 'Aphasic Children'. Volta Bureau, Washington.

Monsees, E. K. (1961). Aphasia in children. *J. Speech Hear. Dis.* **26**, 83–86.

Myklebust, H. R. (1971). Childhood Aphasia. *In* 'Handbook of Speech Pathology and Audiology' (L. E. Travis, ed.), pp. 1181–1202. Appleton-Century-Crofts, New York.

Poppen, R., Stark, J., Eisenson, J., Forrest, T. and Wertheim, G. (1969). Visual sequencing performance of aphasic children. *J. Speech Hear. Res.* **12**, 288–300.

Schlanger, B. and Gottesleben, R. H. (1957). Analysis of speech defects among the institutional mentally retarded. *Training Sch. Bull.* **54**, 5–8.

Stambak, M. (1959). Les audi-mutités. *Psychol. Française* **4**, 146–147.

Stark, J. (1967). A comparison of the performance of aphasic children on three sequencing tests. *J. Comm. Dis.* **1**, 31–34.

Stark, J., Poppen, R. and May, M. Z. (1967). Effects of alterations of prosodic features on the sequencing performance of aphasic children. *J. Speech Hear. Res.* **10**, 849–855.

Swisher, L. and Hirsh, I. J. (1972). Brain damage and the ordering of two temporally successive stimuli. *Neuropsychologia* **10**, 137–152.

Tallal, P. and Piercy, M. (1973a). Defects of non-verbal auditory perception in children with developmental aphasia. *Nature* **241**, 468–469.

Tallal, P. and Piercy, M. (1973b). Developmental aphasia: impaired rate of non-verbal processing as a function of sensory modality. *Neuropsychologia* **11**, 389–398.

Tallal, P. and Piercy, M. (1974). Developmental aphasia: rate of auditory processing and selective impairment of consonant perception. *Neuropsychologia* **12**, 83–93.

Tallal, P. and Piercy, M. (1975). Developmental aphasia: the perception of brief vowels and extended stop consonants. *Neuropsychologia* **13**, 69–74.

Thurrell, R. J. and Josephson, T. S. (1966). Retinoblastoma and intelligence. *Psychosomatics* **7**, 368–370.

Vanderplas, J. M. and Garvin, E. A. (1959). The association value of random shapes. *J. exp. Psychol.* **57**, 147–154.

Weiner, P. (S. 1969). The perceptual level of functioning of dysphasic children. *Cortex* **5**, 440–457.

Wilde, W. (1853). 'Practical Observations on Aural Surgery'. Blanchard and Lea, Philadelphia.

Wiley, J. (1971). A Psychology of Auditory Impairment. *In* 'Psychology of Exceptional Children and Youth' (W. M. Cruickshank, ed.), 3rd edition, pp. 414–439. Prentice Hall, Englewood Cliffs, New Jersey.

Williams, M. (1968). Superior intelligence of children blinded from retino-blastoma. *Arch. Dis. Childh.* **43**, 204–210.

Wilson, L. F., Doehring, D. G. and Hirsh, I. J. (1960). Auditory discrimination learning by aphasic and nonaphasic children. *J. Speech Hear. Res.* **3**, 130–137.

Worster-Drought, C. and Allen, I. M. (1929a). Congenital auditory imperception (congenital word-deafness) with report of case. *J. Neurol. Psychopathol.* **9**, 193–208.

Worster-Drought, C. and Allen, I. M. (1929b). Congenital auditory imperception (congenital word-deafness); investigation of case by Head's method. *J. Neurol. Psychopathol.* **9**, 289–319.

Worster-Drought, C. and Allen, I. M. (1930). Congenital auditory imperception (congenital word-deafness) and its relation to idioglossia and other speech defects. *J. Neurol. Psychopathol.* **10**, 193–236.

Zangwill, O. L. (1964). Intelligence in Aphasia. *In* 'Disorders of Language' (A. V. S. de Reuck and M. O'Connor, eds), pp. 261–274. Little, Brown and Co., Boston.

Defects of Auditory Perception
in Children with
Developmental Dysphasia

Paula Tallal and Malcolm Piercy

Introduction

The failure to develop a particular cognitive skill is almost always more difficult to understand than a comparable defect occurring for the first time in adult life. It is beyond the scope of the present chapter to pursue this question in any detail but two general points may be made by way of introduction to our discussion of developmental anomalies in the perception of language. First, when cognitive deficit occurs in the adult (e.g. as a consequence of cerebral lesion), even though we may not know precisely which mechanism is impaired, the general character of the disability is fairly obvious when compared with pre-morbid performance. With developmental defects, however, there is no pre-morbid performance upon which we can base our deductions. To take a closely relevant example, acquired deafness in the adult will not affect language comprehension as tested by reading. Among the congenitally deaf, however, reading skills are notoriously difficult to acquire owing presumably to the absence of a substrate of spoken language on which reading may be built.

A second difficulty arises from the fact that a particular functional failure may have quite different and more extensive consequences if it is present when postnatal experience begins than if it develops subsequent to the acquisition of a wide range of cognitive skills. There is considerable sensitivity to this problem in cases of dyslexia where, for example, there is widespread suspicion that a degree of spatial imperception, which would not adversely affect reading once the skill is attained, might nonetheless constitute a severe impediment to its acquisition. Because developmental dysphasia is apparent at a much earlier stage of development than dyslexia, difficulties of this kind are perhaps under-emphasised. There is, of course, a general awareness that a wide range of capacities is necessary when learning to speak and to understand speech, but there is also a general presumption that deficits involving these specific components (e.g. sensory, perceptual, intellectual, motor, personality features) may be readily identified. In consequence diagnosis of specific developmental language delay is characteristically diagnosis by exclusion. When everything obvious, apart from a defect of language itself, has been excluded, what remains is, by definition, either a defect intrinsic to language as such, or else something quite unsuspected. If one is interested in the origins of developmental language disability, the choice is in practice between examining linguistic anomalies (as in Paula Menyuk's chapter), and carefully re-examining the components which have been excluded, in case the exclusion has been too gross and undiscriminating. Naturally, the first alternative is the most appealing because it encroaches upon largely unexplored territory and because it can reasonably be construed as a direct examination of the disability as presented. This alternative does, however, carry the disadvantage that whatever high level linguistic disability may be demonstrated, it could in principle be secondary to something simpler. It is the purpose of this chapter to exemplify this second alternative by considering evidence relating to auditory perceptual capacity independently of whether or not the material to be perceived is linguistic in character.

Sensory Defects

As soon as we turn our attention to the possibility that sensory defects may underlie developmental dysphasia, we encounter problems of definition and classification. If developmental dysphasia is in part defined by excluding sensory defects, then we are looking for an explanation where, in logic, none is to be found. The solution to this dilemma is presumably to suspend judgement concerning definition and to accept as criteria for exclusion only those defects whose role in language acquisition is both plausible and reasonably well understood. Thus, there is no cause for excitement in the observation that a totally deaf child has difficulty in learning to acquire language. More subtle sensory defects, however, deserve attention. Indeed, our problem may be defined by asking the question: are there any cases of conventionally diagnosed developmental dysphasia which do not have this particular sensory defect? If the answer to this question turns out to be 'yes', then either the disability we are interested in has more than one sufficient cause, or else we have failed to isolate a key feature of the developmental anomaly. If the experimental answer to the question is 'no', then it is probable that either a necessary cause or a concomitant of a necessary cause has been identified. An example of the first type is provided by Ewing (1930) who showed that six of ten developmental aphasic children had raised thresholds for certain high frequencies. There is now a consensus of opinion that with the improvement of audiometric techniques, the kind of hearing loss identified by Ewing can be excluded before arriving at a diagnosis of developmental dysphasia. At the least, it may be said that the degree of simple peripheral hearing loss of this kind in aphasic children is small, if present at all, and not sufficient to explain the severe language retardation.

Other sensory deficits have been noted in children with language disorders, for example, abnormal auditory temporal summation (Rosenthal, 1971) and masking level differences (Rosenthal and Wohlert, 1973). But the results of these and other psychoacoustic studies, which use pure tone or other simple non-verbal acoustic stimuli, have not been related directly to speech processing. It is known that certain non-verbal and verbal acoustic processing occur, at least in part, in different hemispheres of the brain (see Milner, 1971 for review). Furthermore, studies with hearing-impaired subjects suggest that sensory deficits alone do not necessary entail language disabilities (Danaher and Pickett, 1975).

If we intend to investigate whether impaired auditory mechanisms are causal in language delay, it would seem important to include examination of higher level auditory perceptual processes, which may be directly concerned with speech perception. Clinical descriptions of children with specific developmental language dysfunction have often reported auditory perceptual deficits. Thus Benton (1964), in his original definition of the syndrome 'developmental aphasia', considered that there was evidence suggesting that the basis of the disorder is a high level deficit of auditory perception. Monsees (1957) stressed the possible importance of temporal sequencing deficits in developmental aphasics. Hardy (1965) described the aphasic child's difficulties with what he called 'auding' or 'the integrative functions in the brain's management of auditory information' and suggested that such difficulties may result in the inability to distinguish between similar sounding words. Eisenson, in a series of informative articles on developmental aphasia (1968, 1972) described the types of perceptual impairments which have been observed in most aphasic children. These included: (a) defective capacity for storing speech signals (McReynolds, 1966), (b) impairment of phoneme recognition specifically within contextual utterance, and (c) impairment in processing sequences of speech events at the rate at which they normally occur.

These observations have provided bases for the experimental investigation of the perceptual abilities of dysphasic children. In particular, interest has focused on the role of auditory sequencing and auditory memory.

Experimental Investigations of the Perception of Temporal Sequence in Normal, Dysphasic and Brain Damaged Children

Lowe and Campbell (1965) studied children whom they classified as 'aphasoid' using the methods originally employed by Efron (1963) in the study of perception of temporal order in adult aphasics. In this experiment, 'aphasoids' were compared with normal children, matched for age, on their ability to judge 'succession', i.e., auditory fusion as described by Hirsh (1959): the inter-sound-interval (ISI) at which two stimuli are heard as two sounds rather than one. They were also tested on their ability to judge temporal order. Two different 15 ms pure tones (400 Hz and 2200 Hz) were presented in rapid succession (with brief ISIs) and subjects were required to indicate which of the two tones occurred first. No significant difference between the two groups' performance was demonstrated on the 'succession' task. Compared with the normal controls, however, the 'aphasoid' subjects were significantly impaired in their ability to indicate which of the two tones occurred first when they they were presented in rapid succession. The normal controls made correct temporal order judgements with ISIs at 15 ms to 80 ms (mean = 35·8 ms). The 'aphasoids' required intervals of 55 ms to 700 ms (mean = 357 ms) to achieve the same level of performance as the controls (75 per cent correct). Lowe and Campbell concluded that disturbed temporal ordering might be a major factor in the communication difficulties of 'aphasoid' children.

Aten and Davis (1968) carried out an extensive study of the perception of non-verbal and verbal auditory sequences in children whom they classified as having 'minimal cerebral dysfunction' (MCD). They included children with one or more definite 'signs' of central nervous system disorder in their MCD group. Evidence of central nervous system disorder included abnormal electroencephalogram, seizures, head injuries and bilateral haematomas. Their tests of non-verbal auditory perception included (a) reproducing rhythmically presented sequences of pure tones and (b) judging the duration of pure tone sound bursts by selecting a short, medium, or long plastic block corresponding in length to the relative duration of the tone. The tests of verbal perception included (a) serial memory span for nonsense syllables, digits and words, (b) verbal reproduction of multi-syllabic words presented sequentially, scrambled sentences, and paragraphs. In general, the performance of the MCD group was poorer than that of the control group on perceptual memory span and number of stimuli accurately reproduced. The MCD group was most impaired on auditory stimuli which varied in rhythm and duration.

This evidence suggests that perception, storage and reproduction of sequential auditory stimuli may be disturbed by cerebral dysfunction.

Griffiths (1972) reported a study in which developmental aphasic and normal children were tested for their ability to reproduce non-verbal rhythmic patterns. Rhythmic patterns were tapped in 4/4, 6/8, and 3/4 time on a tambourine within the child's vision at the rate of approximately two crochets (quarter notes) per second. The subjects were required to reproduce the pattern immediately on another tambourine. Although the aphasic children performed as well as control subjects on the simplest patterns (showing that they understood the task) they were markedly impaired when reproducing the more complex rhythmic patterns. Griffiths suggested that difficulties in temporal ordering of auditory stimuli, discrimination of relative duration or memory span could be responsible for the impaired performance of the developmental aphasics at this task.

Monsees (1968) studied the ability of children with 'expressive' language disorders and normal controls to (a) repeat isolated phonemes presented over a loudspeaker (thus eliminating visual cues), (b) make same-different judgements on pairs of nonsense syllables (Templin Sound Discrimination Test, Templin 1957), (c) 'blend' a sequence of phonemes into a word (for example, /p/+/ai/ = /pai/) and (d) repeat a sequence of phonemes in the order of their presentation. The results showed no significant difference between the abilities of the children with and without 'expressive' language disorders to imitate isolated phonemes. The performance of the language-impaired group, however, was significantly inferior to that of the controls on all other tasks studied. This study provided evidence that the previously reported inability of dysphasics and other language-impaired children to report the temporal order of non-verbal auditory stimuli, as might be expected, also applies to verbal stimuli.

Poppen et al. (1969) point out that several authors have reported not only auditory perceptual impairments in developmental dysphasic children, but also visual perceptual and visual memory impairments (Stark, 1966, 1967; Furth and Pufall, 1966; Withrow, 1964). These authors investigated sequencing abilities of aphasic, deaf and normal children. They found that, whereas there was no difference between the aphasic and deaf children in their studies, both of these groups of children were inferior to normal control children on tasks requiring them to reproduce a temporal, spatial sequence of visual stimuli. Poppen et al. (1969) suggest that aphasic children exhibit similar impairments in both the auditory and the visual modality on sequencing tests, and hence they have a *general* sequencing deficit which may underlie their language impairment. It should be emphasised, however, that this conclusion could only be drawn if the visual stimuli and the auditory stimuli in the sequencing tests studied had been presented in the same manner, either both spatially or both temporally. This was not the case in these experiments.

The experiments investigating the auditory and the visual sequencing abilities of dysphasic children have suggested that these children may have both auditory temporal sequencing deficits and visual temporal, spatial sequencing deficits. These experiments, however, have been few in number, have utilised different criteria for inclusion of subjects into the experimental groups and have also employed different experimental paradigms. Furthermore, the relationship between the severity of impairment in sequencing experiments and the severity of language impairment in dysphasic children has not been investigated.

A weakness common to all of the sequencing experiments so far reviewed is the failure to show that subjects were able to discriminate accurately between two stimulus elements when they were combined and presented rapidly in succession. In every experiment reported it had been assumed that because discrimination between stimulus elements presented in isolation had been demonstrated, deficits in perception of rapidly presented sequences composed of these elements must be the result of a failure to perceive temporal order. Hirsh (1959), however, pointed out that, in order to perceive accurately the sequence of a rapidly-presented two-element stimulus pair, one must perceive the two elements as separate rather than fused and then decide whether they are the same or different. Nevertheless, in subsequent experiments designed to assess sequencing ability, various authors failed to ensure that subjects could perform these more primary perceptual tasks. It is possible, therefore, that at rapid rates of stimulus presentation, subjects had difficulty in discriminating between the various stimuli, although having no difficulty in discrimination at slower rates of presentation. Poor performance on tests of perception of temporal order would then occur in consequence and the possibility of a sequencing deficit would not have been examined. This could apply to any experiment which investigated perception of temporal order in language-impaired children and failed to control for accuracy in the discrimination of rapidly presented stimuli.

Sequencing experiments with language-impaired subjects have also been criticised on other grounds. Rees (1973) emphasised three particular problems which introduce difficulties in interpretation. First, theories based on results of studies in which pure tones have been used as stimuli can be criticised on the grounds that pure tones may be processed differently from speech sounds (Kimura, 1967; Milner, 1971). Second, it may be argued that studies which have used verbal stimuli to assess the perceptual abilities of language-disordered subjects confound the effects of perception and linguistic ability. Impairment observed in such studies may simply reflect a disorder of language. Finally, investigators have failed to establish a positive correlation between the extent of perceptual sequencing disorder in language-impaired subjects and the extent of their impairment of language.

Rees concluded that even if a primary perceptual difficulty were isolated in language-delayed children, there would still be little evidence to suggest that it is systematically related to the language disability.

We felt that, to understand the relationship between basic perceptual disorders and language delay, a new experimental method was required. Thus, we sought a means of generating non-verbal stimuli which 'imitated' the acoustic properties of steady-state speech sounds, such as vowels, but did not match the acoustic spectrum of any specific phoneme. Such signals could be acoustically 'speech-like' whilst at the same time being linguistically meaningless. Recent work in psychoacoustics, together with the development of speech synthesisers, has made it possible to specify and generate the acoustic features which define such signals.

In order to explore the perceptual deficits of children with language disorder, it was also necessary to devise a method which would enable subjects to report non-verbally, yet in detail, exactly what they perceived at each stimulus presentation. Similarly, it was important that the method should be easily demonstrable without the need of verbal instruction or verbal response. We needed an experimental procedure which permitted the examination of various aspects of perception in a uniform fashion so that results obtained in studies using non-verbal complex acoustic stimuli could be directly compared with results from similar studies using non-verbal visual stimuli, and with results from similar studies using verbal stimuli.

In the experiments discussed below, a non-verbal operant conditioning method was used, designed to meet the above requirements. This method was labelled the 'Repetition Method' and has been described in detail in a previous publication (Tallal and Piercy, 1973b). In each experiment, whether auditory or visual, verbal or non-verbal, the same general experimental procedure was used. Subjects were trained to respond by pressing on two identical panels mounted side by side. Each panel corresponded to one of two stimuli and, when these stimuli were presented successively, a corresponding sequence of panel presses was required (i.e. 1, 1; 1, 2; 2, 1; 2, 2). In the first instance, the demands on auditory processing were manipulated by varying the duration of the inter-stimulus interval (ISI) between two complex tones which did not correspond to particular phonemes but whose frequencies were within the speech range. The duration of the tones was held constant at 75 ms. The dysphasic children when compared with normal children (matched for age, sex and non-verbal intelligence) were impaired when the ISI was shortened to 150 ms or less. These results are, of course, consistent with earlier suggestions that dysphasic children have a sequencing deficit, i.e. difficulty in perceiving and responding to temporal order.

In a different version of this experiment, however, the same subjects were trained to press one panel when the two stimuli were the same (i.e. 1,1 or 2, 2) and the other panel when they were different (i.e. 1, 2 or 2, 1). Using this same-different technique, we found that the dysphasic children were just as impaired as they were with the 'repetition' technique. Because the same-different procedure (unlike the repetition technique) does not demand perception of temporal order, only perception of identity or difference, we concluded that, when the ISI was short, our children with language disorders were impaired in their ability to discriminate the two tones. Similarly, because they were equally impaired on the repetition and the same-different procedures, we concluded that the apparent sequencing difficulty on the repetition task could be regarded as entirely secondary to the defect of discrimination. Given these results, the frequently reported sequencing defect shown by other studies of developmental dysphasia must be questioned. In the absence of evidence to the contrary, it would seem justifiable to attribute these reported difficulties in perceiving the temporal order of auditory stimuli to a failure to discriminate the sound quality of the stimuli when these are presented in rapid succession.

Having established that our subjects with developmental dysphasia failed to discriminate two different complex tones when the ISI was reduced, we tested for a comparable deficit in the visual modality. Substituting different coloured lights (two shades of green) for the auditory stimuli but replicating the temporal characteristics of the auditory experiment, we found no significant differences between the dysphasic and the control groups (Tallal and Piercy, 1973b). In the dysphasic children the defect observed was therefore specific to the auditory modality. Yet a number of authors have reported that dysphasic children have difficulty in sequencing visual as well as auditory material. Two considerations are relevant here. First, studies which claimed a defect with visual stimuli introduced further complications. For instance, in some studies visual sequences were presented spatially as well as temporally, whereas in our test the visual temporal sequences were always presented at a single spatial location. Also, other studies used a delayed reaction procedure, whereas our subjects were free to respond as soon as the stimulus pattern was completed. It is possible that confounding spatial and temporal sequences and enforcing a delay in response placed a premium on verbal mediation, to the disadvantage of the dysphasic children.

The second consideration concerns the criteria used in selecting dysphasic children. Variations in these criteria may have resulted in different investigators studying different types of dysphasic children. In our study, for example, the only children included in the dysphasic group were those with normal non-verbal intelligence as measured by Raven's Coloured Progressive Matrices (Raven, 1962). The implementation of this criterion may have resulted in the exclusion of dysphasic children with visual perceptual impairment. Equally, we cannot claim that our children were unimpaired on tasks involving spatial sequencing because we did not examine such performances. What we can say, however, is that the dysphasic children showed a defect in auditory discrimination which did not have a counterpart in the visual modality.

The adverse effect of short ISIs on the dysphasic children's performance on the auditory task was not absolute; it could be compensated for by increasing the duration of the stimuli. Indeed, it became clear that it was the total duration of the two stimuli and the interval between them that was critical for the performance of the dysphasic children. In these experiments, the two-element sound pattern consisted of tone 1, ISI, tone 2; and the duration of the ISI and of the tone were varied independently in different experimental conditions. We found that the total time between the onset of tone 1 and the 'offset' of tone 2 correlated significantly with the dysphasic children's performance (rho = 0·89). It was therefore suggested that the dysphasic children were unable to perceive acoustic information accurately when it was presented at a rapid rate, and it seemed possible that this constraint on speed of auditory processing might underlie their language impairment.

Auditory Processing and Speech Perception

A brief consideration of some of the recent work on speech synthesis and comprehension yields some clues as to how such a defect of auditory processing might affect language comprehension. At a relatively superficial level, a radical distinction may be made between the acoustic properties of vowels and of certain consonants. The essential cue for the perception of vowels is the steady-state frequencies of the first three formants which are of relatively long duration (e.g. 250 ms). The essential cue for stop-consonants differs from that for vowels in two important respects: it is briefer in duration (c. 50 ms) and the critical formants are not steady-state but transitional in character, the component frequencies changing rapidly with time (Fry et al., 1962; Liberman et al., 1957). These considerations alone would justify examining the ability of dysphasic children to perceive vowels and stop-consonants. There are, however, other equally important considerations.

It has been pointed out (Liberman et al., 1957) that two remarkable features of speech perception are the rate at which speech can be perceived and the accuracy with which information relating to temporal order is retained. Speech can be comprehended without temporal order confusions at some 400 words/min or approximately 30 phonemes/s (Orr *et al.*, 1965). This far exceeds human temporal resolving power for non-verbal stimuli (Hirsh, 1959). It has also been shown (Liberman *et al.*, 1957) that, when certain syllables are perceived, there is not an invariant correspondence between phonemes and sound spectrum. Rather, information concerning successive phonemes is transmitted simultaneously throughout the duration of the syllable. The shape, combination and distribution of transients are evidently crucial in determining the perception of complex, rapidly transmitted sequences of phonemes. Dorman *et al.* (1975) showed that perception of the temporal order of sequences of phonemes is far superior in running speech than in concatenated speech consisting of vowel series without transitions. These authors conclude that one of the higher level functions of formant transitions is to bind together sequences of phonemes so that the temporal order of speech sounds may be preserved even at rapid rates of transmission (see also Cole and Scott, 1973). At least three important functions, therefore, have reasonably been claimed for formant transitions: the mediation of certain phonemes; 'parallel' transmission of phonemes constituting syllables; and the binding together of speech segments in running speech.

From this brief discussion, it may be seen that an inability to perceive phonemes mediated by formant transitions might have far-reaching consequences in language development. Accordingly, our twelve dysphasic children and the matched normal controls were tested, using the experimental procedures described above, for their ability to discriminate (*a*) between two synthesised steady-state vowels and (*b*) between two synthesised stop-consonants (Tallal and Piercy, 1974). The first of these experiments used synthesised versions of the vowels /ɛ/ and /ae/, each of 250 ms duration, i.e. the duration at which (on the basis of a previous experiment) the dysphasic children, as well as the controls, could discriminate between non-verbal complex tones at all ISIs studied. The results were quite clear-cut. Both groups of children could discriminate between the synthesised vowels at all ISIs as efficiently as they had discriminated between the two non-verbal stimuli. No significant differences between groups were observed on any task studied using the vowel stimuli. Clearly the performance of the dysphasic children did not deteriorate when vowels were substituted for complex tones which did not correspond to phonemes. But, of course, both of these classes of stimuli were of a steady-state character.

The next experiment employed the synthesised stop-consonants /ba/ and /da/, each of 250 ms total duration. These stimuli are more accurately described as consonant-vowel syllables because both terminate with the same steady-state vowel and the discriminable components last for only 40 ms and consist of the initial formant transitions characteristic of the consonants. The experiment was replicated with these stimuli following the procedure described above. On all tasks studied the performance of the dysphasic children was significantly inferior to that of the normal controls. Furthermore, the performance of the dysphasic children with these stimuli was significantly inferior to their own performance with vowels and with non-verbal stimuli.

The synthesised consonants differed from the vowel stimuli in two respects: the discriminable components were of shorter duration; and the stimuli to be discriminated consisted of acoustic information which was transitional in character, not steady-state. Two further experiments established the relative importance of these differences (Tallal and Piercy, 1975). First, performance was examined on two diphthong-like vowel-vowel syllables, which possessed the following characteristics: (a) the first and second part of each stimulus were respectively of the same duration as the first and second part of the consonant-vowel syllables already described; (b) all the acoustic information was steady-state in character (there was a straight cut between the first and second components of each stimulus); (c) the second part of both stimuli was identical; (d) both stimuli were of 250 ms total duration. In other words, the temporal features of the original consonant experiment were preserved but no transitions were employed. The vowel-vowel stimuli used synthesised versions of /ɛI/ and /aeI/. When these stimuli were used, the performance of the dysphasic children was the same on all tasks studied as their performance on the consonant experiment, i.e. they were grossly impaired in comparison with the controls. This established that the brevity of the discriminable component of the consonant stimuli was sufficient to result in impaired discrimination by the dysphasic children.

These results did not, however, exclude the possibility that the dysphasic children were impaired in perceiving and discriminating between transients as such, in addition to their difficulties in processing acoustic information which was brief in duration. To test this, a second experiment was carried out. The formant transitions of the synthesised consonant-vowel stimuli were extended from 40 ms to 80 ms while maintaining the total duration of each stimulus at 250 ms by reducing the duration of the steady-state component common to the two stimuli. Thus the discriminable component of each stimulus was increased in duration from 40 ms to 80 ms but this component remained transitional in character. Using these stimuli, there were no significant differences between the performance of the dysphasic and the normal children in any of the tasks studied. It is notable that the normal children continued to perceive these stimuli as /ba/ and /da/ (see Tallal, 1977). The dysphasic children could therefore discriminate between speech sounds mediated by transitions provided they were sufficiently long in duration.

We have suggested that a failure to discriminate between different rapid formant transitions might well have disruptive effects on language acquisition over and above the ability to discriminate between consonants which are mediated by particular transitions occurring in a specified vowel context. Nonetheless, if developmental dysphasia stems from failure to perceive particular speech sounds, then it would be predicted that these same speech sounds would be omitted or produced incorrectly by the dysphasic children. This prediction was tested (Tallal *et al.*, 1976) with the same group of children who served as subjects in the previous experiments.

Relationship between Speech Perception and Speech Production

These twelve dysphasic children and matched normal controls were tested for their ability to imitate (*a*) isolated steady-state vowels such as /ɛ/ and /ae/ (these are not the same as vowels in word context, which rarely reach the steady-state spectral pattern we are describing here), (*b*) stop-consonants in consonant-vowel nonsense syllables (e.g. /bɛ/ and /dɛ/), (*c*) stop-consonants in consonant-vowel-consonant nonsense syllables (e.g. /bɛk/ and /dɛg/) and (*d*) stop-consonants in clusters (e.g. /blɛ/ and /prɛ/). All categories of sound were produced by the examiner. The subjects were also required to produce the names of pictures of objects shown individually on cards. The names of the objects were words of a single syllable comprising stop-consonants in the initial and final position (e.g. bed, cup), as well as words comprising primarily vowels (e.g. eye, ear), diphthongs and nasals (knife, nose). All the subjects' responses were recorded on magnetic tape and later transcribed phonetically by two independent listeners.

The data were analysed in terms of the overall percentage of errors made on isolated vowels, nasals, stop-consonants, both singly and in clusters, occurring in the speech sample. The results showed that the normal children were able to produce isolated vowels, nasals, stop-consonants and consonant-clusters equally well. In the case of the dysphasic children, while the production of isolated vowels was within normal limits, their production of stop-consonants both singly and in clusters was grossly impaired.

The relationship between impairment of speech perception and impairment of speech production is also evident when sub-groups of the dysphasic children are compared. Of the group studied in the perceptual experiments, five of the twelve subjects were *unimpaired* in their discrimination of stop-consonants presented singly rather than in sequences of two. The remaining seven subjects were unable to discriminate these phonemes, even when presented singly. The speech production performance of the dysphasic children was analysed in terms of their perceptual performance. The perceptually 'unimpaired' group performed as well as normal control subjects on the production of isolated vowels and stop-consonants. They were also normal in their production of nasals (although the *perception* of nasals has not been investigated). When the production of stop-consonants in clusters was required, however, their performance was significantly impaired.

The performance of the perceptually 'impaired' group of dysphasics was significantly worse than that of the perceptually 'unimpaired' group on all four measures of speech production studied. Furthermore, their pattern of impairment corresponded to their perceptual impairment: i.e. the production of isolated vowels and nasals was significantly less impaired than that of stop-consonants, particularly in clusters.

These findings suggest that the speech production deficits of these dysphasic children mirror their defects of speech perception. Those speech sounds incorporating rapid spectral changes critical for their perception are most difficult for dysphasic children to perceive and are also most often inaccurately produced. These results add further support to the hypothesis that developmental dysphasia can be accounted for, at least in part, by a failure to develop an auditory perceptual process necessary for the perception of speech.

Serial Memory Performance

The results so far described are most easily understood as a failure to make perceptual use of acoustic information which is very brief in duration and rapidly changing. We have suggested that there may be a constraint on the speed at which such information can be processed. However, our dysphasic children (and the controls) were also given tasks which are better described as tests of serial memory than perceptual tests, and the interpretation of these results is less straightforward. In the case of non-verbal complex tones, vowels and consonants, all subjects were tested, using the repetition method, for their ability to respond appropriately to binary sequences consisting of three, four and five elements (e.g. 1, 2, 1; 2, 1, 2, 1; 1, 1, 2, 2, 1). The interval between successive elements in a sequence was constant at 428 ms.

When the stimuli were consonant-vowel syllables with a discriminable component of only 40 ms, the dysphasic children performed, not surprisingly, significantly worse than controls irrespective of the number of elements in the sequence. This is consistent with what was observed with two-element patterns. However, the performance of dysphasic children on serial memory tasks involving the two synthesised vowel stimuli introduces a complication. It may be remembered that, when tested with these steady-state, 250 ms stimuli, no significant differences were observed between the ability of dysphasic and control subjects to respond appropriately to two-element patterns, with either short or long ISIs. The same can also be said for serial memory performance with long ISIs involving either 3 or 4 elements. However, when tested on 5-element patterns (the elements being vowels) the dysphasic children were impaired in comparison with the controls. Because the sequences presented and the intervals between them were both of long duration, two interpretations are possible. First, in addition to the perceptual defect already demonstrated, the dysphasic children may also have defective memory for the temporal order of auditory stimuli (i.e. a sequencing defect) when the sequence is relatively long. Alternatively, it could be argued that dysphasic children need disproportionately more time to process longer sequences. Although the second alternative has the advantage of maintaining theoretical consistency (by invoking the concept of speed of processing), it has the disadvantage of making additional assumptions.

Nonetheless, evidence relevant to the second alternative is provided by serial memory performance for non-verbal complex tones. In these experiments (Tallal and Piercy, 1973b) the same long ISI (428 ms) was employed as for serial memory with vowels and consonants but the effect of two different tone durations was studied: 250 ms (as for the vowels and consonants) and 75 ms. With tone durations of 250 ms, dysphasic subjects performed slightly more poorly than they did with vowel stimuli. With non-verbal tones they performed at a significantly lower level than controls not only on 5-element patterns (as they did with the vowel stimuli) but also on 4-element patterns. It is notable that this result cannot be attributed to a greater acoustic difference between the two vowel stimuli than between the two non-verbal stimuli. It seems therefore that, once dysphasic children can perceive speech sounds accurately they, like normal subjects (Miller, 1967), can use verbal mediation to improve their serial memory span.

On the 2-element non-verbal task, dysphasic children performed as well as controls when the ISI was 428 ms and the tone duration was 75 ms. Yet with the same stimuli and the same ISI, dysphasic children performed significantly more poorly than controls on serial memory for sequences of 3, 4 and 5 elements (p < ·001 in each case). No such differences were observed with visual stimuli conforming to the same temporal patterns. The dysphasic children's serial memory performance is improved, however, when the duration of the tones is increased. They perform significantly better with 250 ms stimuli than with 75 ms stimuli on 3- and 4-element patterns (there is a floor effect on 5-element patterns).

The hypothesis that dysphasic children need disproportionately more time to process longer sequences gains, therefore, some support from these findings. Within certain limits, this proposition accurately describes the performance of the dysphasic children in comparison with normal controls when ISI is held constant and tone duration and number of elements are varied. On 2-element patterns with tone durations of 75 ms, dysphasic children perform as well as controls but on 3-element patterns they perform significantly more poorly. Yet, increasing tone duration to 250 ms removes the difference between dysphasics and controls on 3-element patterns.

Although this evidence concerning serial memory in relation to stimulus duration lends plausibility to the notion that the impairment shown by dysphasic children on tests of auditory serial memory may be reduced to defective speed of auditory processing, the possibility that there is an additional independent defect of memory for temporal order is a strong one. It is entirely possible that the advantage conferred on the serial memory of dysphasic children when tone duration is increased has an exact counterpart in normal children. If this were the case, the effect in dysphasic children would argue neither for nor against the 'speed of processing' hypothesis. Unfortunately, in the context of the experiments described, a ceiling effect makes it impossible to decide with any confidence whether or not such an effect occurs in normal children. It is, however, a question which further experiment could answer.

Whatever the underlying cause, dysphasic children do *in effect* have inferior memory for auditory sequences and evidence, even among the children serving as subjects in these experiments, is not confined to the special test procedures described. The same children were examined on the Token Test devised by De Renzi and Vignolo (1962) to examine the receptive abilities of adult aphasics. Tallal (1975) showed that the dysphasic children had little difficulty in recognising familiar words which are very different from each other acoustically, provided these words are presented singly. They experience considerable difficulty, however, in responding appropriately to commands which combine these words, in sequence. In a developmental study Whitaker and Noll (1972) showed that most normal children make progressively more errors on consecutive sections of the Token Test, most errors occurring on Part 5 which is marked by greater grammatical complexity than earlier parts. Part 4, on the other hand, is characterised by a greater load of adjectival information in the object noun phrases, thus making greater demands on verbal memory. The dysphasic children performed more poorly than controls on Parts 2, 3, 4 and 5 but their poorest performance was on Part

4 (as was the performance of the 12 controls). Furthermore, the errors of the dysphasic children on Part 5 were of a particular type: there was a tendency to respond only to the concluding phrase of a complex command. Thus the response to 'If there is a black circle, pick up the red square' (the black circle being absent) tended to be incorrect and the response to 'Instead of the white square, take the yellow circle' tended to be correct. It appeared that, although the dysphasic children performed much more poorly than the controls throughout the test, they were especially vulnerable to demands on auditory memory but, within the constraints of this disability, were not disproportionately vulnerable to grammatical complexity.

Relationship between Auditory Defect and Linguistic Defect

There is of course no suggestion that the dysphasic children whose performance we have described have no difficulties with grammatical aspects of language. They quite obviously do have such difficulties. What is at issue in the present context is whether there is a primary linguistic defect or whether much or all of their language deficits stems from the auditory perceptual defects with which we have been concerned. We would suggest that these perceptual deficits constitute a *prima facie* case for a reductionist position in relation to developmental dysphasia. It remains, however, to consider first the evidence derived from studies showing specific linguistic deficits on children with developmental dysphasia; and second how, in principle, we might arrive, through experiment, at a decision concerning any causal relationship, between the auditory perceptual defect and the linguistic disability.

Two studies are representative of the difficulties in reaching decisions concerning the nature of developmental dysphasia by investigating linguistic aspects of performance. In one study Morehead and Ingram (1973) collected language samples and wrote grammars for linguistically deviant and normal children. Five aspects of syntactic development were chosen for a comparison between the two groups: phrase structure rules, transformations, construction (or sentence) types, inflectional morphology, and minor lexical categories. Few significant differences between groups were found for learning the more general aspects of syntax. The only significant qualitative differences between the groups were found in the use of infrequently occurring transformations and in the number of major syntactic categories per construction type. The major difference between the groups appeared to be quantitative in character; the deviant group showed a marked delay in the onset of and acquisition time for learning base syntax.

In another study, Hughes (1972) trained aphasic children to use a symbolic system similar to that reported by Premack (1971) to teach chimpanzees to communicate. Hughes used a number of meaningless shapes to serve as symbols which could be moved about on a magnetic board. She was able to teach the children to use the shapes as signs for particular objects and, in addition, was able to teach them a number of language functions, such as direct and indirect objects, negation, modifiers and questions. The language-impaired children were not only able to use the system to perform a number of generalisation tests, but were also able to manipulate the shapes so as to produce new utterances. Within a ten week training period, the language-impaired children were able to learn to use these symbols to communicate, by-passing the auditory modality.

Neither of these studies suggests that the linguistic abilities of children with developmental dysphasia are qualitatively rather than quantitatively different from those of normal children. Equally they cannot be said to provide convincing evidence to the contrary. For example, Glass et al. (1973) suggest that, within limits, adult global aphasics may be trained to use an artificial language and that the right hemisphere as well as the left may possess the basic cognitive skills necessary for language, although lacking the specialised systems used for the production and understanding of a natural language. Although their patients did not seem to have achieved the communicative facility of the children studied by Hughes, if their suggestion is in principle correct, we would none the less scarcely wish to argue from this that adult aphasics do not have a specifically linguistic defect. By the same token, we might hesitate to say that Hughes has demonstrated that dysphasic children have no primary linguistic deficit.

How then should the demonstration of an auditory perceptual deficit in a group of children with developmental dysphasia be evaluated as a potential explanation of the language disability?

Whilst it is true that we have described a number of experimental results which confirm the hypothesis suggested by our earliest experiments (Tallal and Piercy, 1973a), it is now appropriate to consider which observations would constitute disproof. At the same time we may usefully consider what observations would constitute disproof of alternative hypotheses. There are at least four possible ways in which the presenting disorder of language in cases of developmental dysphasia might be related to our observations of impaired auditory perception (perhaps together with impaired auditory memory). (a) The auditory defect might be a necessary cause of developmental dysphasia; (b) the auditory defect might be a sufficient but not necessary cause of developmental dysphasia; (c) defective auditory perception (and memory) might be secondary to a primary linguistic defect; (d) the auditory defect might be a concomitant of the linguistic defect but not causally related to it. If some of these possibilities could be experimentally excluded then the status of the auditory defect in relation to developmental dysphasia should become considerably clearer.

THE AUDITORY DEFICIT AS A NECESSARY CAUSE
OF DEVELOPMENTAL DYSPHASIA

This notion is, of course, the most extreme theoretical position that could be adopted. This would entail all cases of developmental dysphasia manifesting the auditory defect and would be refuted by the observation of a single case of developmental dysphasia who performed normally at least on our non-verbal perceptual tests. Failure to find such a case would not, of course, constitute strong evidence in favour of the hypothesis because it would be equally consistent with the auditory defect being an inevitable consequence of restricted linguistic experience. Similarly, it would be consistent with the two types of defect being necessarily associated but not causally related. This state of affairs illustrates the well known principle that instances which refute a hypothesis are logically more powerful than instances which confirm a hypothesis.

If it is reasonable to infer that a defect of rapid auditory processing is not more unfavourable to language development than severe or total deafness, then there is a further possible observation which would disprove the hypothesis we are considering. This would involve a comparison between the kind of dysphasic children we have studied and children born with severe deafness. Provided there was no important difference between the two groups in their non-verbal intelligence and, what is perhaps more important, the way they have been educated, then, according to the hypothesis, the deaf children should have at least as much difficulty in developing language as children with developmental dysphasia. If a study of linguistic performances not involving the understanding of spoken language revealed a clear-cut linguistic defect which was not shared with the deaf children then the hypothesis would be disproved. Comparisons could be made either using a suitable sign language, or a system of communication of the type employed by Premack, or else written productions.

THE AUDITORY DEFECT AS A SUFFICIENT CAUSE
OF DEVELOPMENTAL DYSPHASIA

If the auditory defect were a sufficient but not necessary cause of developmental dysphasia this would entail that there was at least one other sufficient cause of developmental language impairment, and cases of developmental dysphasia without the auditory perceptual deficit would be expected. However, all children who learnt to speak and to understand spoken language normally should be free of the defect of auditory processing and, if some children were observed who had developed language normally but who showed a defect of auditory processing of the kind and severity which we have observed in children with developmental dysphasia, then the hypothesis would be refuted.

THE AUDITORY DEFECT SECONDARY TO A PRIMARY LINGUISTIC DEFECT

If the auditory defect were an inevitable consequence of a defect which was primarily linguistic in origin, then all cases of developmental dysphasia should also exhibit the auditory processing defect and a case which did not would refute the hypothesis. However, if it were the case that a primary linguistic defect present from birth increased the probability of a defect of non-verbal auditory processing but did not make it inevitable, then developmental dysphasia in the absence of a defect of auditory processing could not refute such probabilistic hypotheses. Very similar considerations apply to the notion that the defect of auditory processing is causal in developmental dysphasia only in a probabalistic fashion. If such were the case, the auditory defect would be neither a sufficient nor a necessary cause of the dysphasia and the kind of logic which is being considered here would not apply.

THE AUDITORY DEFECT AS A NON-CAUSAL CONCOMITANT OF A LINGUISTIC DEFECT

The possibility that the auditory defect is a concomitant of developmental dysphasia, but not causally related to it, could be directly refuted only if it were postulated that the auditory defect was a *necessary* concomitant. This would be disproved by a case of developmental dysphasia which did not show the defect of auditory processing.

It may well be that developmental dysphasia can be caused in more than one way. The fact that all of our dysphasic children showed the defect on auditory perception does not argue against this, first because the number of subjects tested was small and second because the dysphasic children investigated were a highly selected group. The relatively high non-verbal intelligence of our subjects has already been mentioned. Other selective factors – some possibly quite unsuspected – may well stem from the policy of the school in deciding which children to accept from among those seeking a place, and also from sources determining which children are brought to the attention of a particular school. These considerations render some of the possibilities discussed above more likely than others.

The least likely is the possibility that the auditory perceptual defect is a necessary and sufficient cause of developmental dysphasia.

Although we have discussed a number of hypotheses relating to the role of the auditory defect in developmental dysphasia, this outline is not exhaustive because probabalistic (as opposed to absolute) relationships have not been covered. Furthermore, because no one can forsee the course of future research the problem of the origins of developmental dysphasia may well eventually be resolved in ways which are at present quite unexpected. Meanwhile, as a stimulus to research we retain our working hypothesis that *some* cases of developmental dysphasia are the direct consequence of defective processing of rapidly changing acoustic information and an associated, possibly consequential reduced memory span for auditory sequence.

Acknowledgements

Thanks are due to the American Association of University Women, Cecil and Ida Green, the Grant Foundation of New York, the Medical Research Council of Great Britain (grant no. G973/144/C) and the National Institute of Health (NINCDS Contract no. 75–09) for their generous support of much of the research described in this chapter.

References

Aten, J. and Davis, J. (1968). Disturbances in the perception of auditory sequence in children with minimal cerebral dysfunction. *J. Speech Hear. Res.* 11, 236–245.

Benton, A. L. (1964). Developmental aphasia and brain damage. *Cortex* 1, 40–52.

Cole, R. A. and Scott, B. (1973). Perception of temporal order in speech; The role of vowel transitions. *Canad. J. Psychol.* 27, 441–449.

Danaher, E. M. and Pickett, J. M. (1975). Some masking effects produced by low frequency vowel formants in persons with sensorineural loss. *J. Speech Hear. Res.* 18, 261–271.

De Renzi, E. and Vignolo, L. A. (1962). Latent sensory aphasia in hemisphere-damage patients: an experimental study with the Token Test. *Brain* 89, 815–830.

Dorman, M. F., Cutting, J. E. and Raphael, L. J. (1975). Perception of temporal order in vowel sequences with and without formant transitions. *J. Exp. Psychol.* Human Perception and Performance. 104, 121–129.

Efron, R. (1963). Temporal perception, aphasia and déjà-vu. *Brain* 86, 403–424.

Eisenson, J. (1968). Developmental aphasia; a speculative view with therapeutic implications. *J. Speech Hear. Dis.* 33 (1), 3–13.

Eisenson, J. (1972). 'Aphasia in Children'. Harper and Row, London.

Ewing, A. G. (1930). 'Aphasia in Children'. Oxford University Press, London.

Fry, D. B., Abramson, A. S., Eimas, P. D. and Liberman, A. M. (1962). The identification and discrimination of synthetic vowels. *Lang. Speech* **5**, 171–188.

Furth, H. G. and Pufall, P. B. (1966). Visual and auditory sequence learning in hearing-impaired children. *J. Speech Hear. Res.* **9**, 441–449.

Glass, A. V., Gazzaniga, M. S. and Premack, D. (1973). Artificial training in global aphasics. *Neuropsychologia* ii, 95–103.

Griffiths, P. (1972). 'Developmental Aphasia; An Introduction'. Invalid Children Aid Association, London.

Hardy, W. G. (1965). On language disorders in young children. A reorganization of thinking. *J. Speech Hear. Res.* **8**, 3–16.

Hirsh, I. J. (1959). Auditory perception of temporal order. *J. Acous. Soc. America.* **31**, 759–767.

Hughes, J. (1972). 'Language and communication; Acquisition of a non-vocal "language" by previously languageless children'. Unpublished Bachelor of Technology thesis, Brunel University, London.

Kimura, D. (1967). Functional asymmetry of the brain in dichotic listening. *Cortex* **3**, 163–178.

Liberman, A. M., Harris, K. S., Hoffman, H. S. and Griffith, B. C. (1957). The discrimination of speech sounds within and across phoneme boundaries. *J. Exp. Psychol.* **54**, 358–368.

Lowe, A. D. and Campbell, R. A. (1965). Temporal discrimination in aphasoid and normal children. *J. Speech Hear. Res.* **8**, 313–314.

McReynolds, L. V. (1966). Operant conditioning for investigating speech sound discrimination in aphasic children. *J. Speech Hear. Res.* **9**, 519–528.

Miller, G. A. (1967). 'The Psychology of Communication – Seven Essays'. Penguin, London.

Milner, B. (1971). Interhemispheric differences in the localisation of psychological processes in man. *Br. Med. Bull.* **27**, 272–277.

Monsees, E. K. (1957). Aphasia in children; diagnosis and education. *Volta Review* **59**, 392–414.

Monsees, E. K. (1968). Temporal sequencing and expressive language disorders. *Excep. Child.* **35** (2), 141–147.

Morehead, D. M. and Ingram, D. (1973). The development of base syntax in normal and linguistically deviant children. *J. Speech Hear. Res.* **16**, 330–352.

Orr, D. B., Friedman, H. L. and Williams, J. C. (1965). Trainability of listening comprehension of speeded discourse. *J. Ed. Psychol.* **56**, 148–156.

Poppen, R., Stark, J., Eisenson, J., Forrest, T. and Wertheim, G. (1969). Visual sequencing performance of aphasic children. *J. Speech Hear. Res.* **12**, 288–300.

Premack, D. (1971). Language in chimpanzee? *Science* **172**, 808–822.

Raven, J. C. (1962). 'Coloured Progressive Matrices'. H. K. Lewis and Co. Ltd, London.

Rees, N. S. (1973). Auditory processing factors in language disorders; The view from Procrustes' bed. *J. Speech Hear. Dis.* **38**, 304–315.

Rosenthal, W. S. (1971). 'Auditory Threshold-Duration Function in Aphasic Subjects; Implications for the Interaction of Linguistic and Auditory Processing in Aphasia'. Paper presented at the 47th annual convention of the American Speech and Hearing Association, Chicago, November 1971.

Rosenthal, W. S. and Wohlert, K. L. (1973). 'Masking Level Differences (MLD) Effects in Aphasic Children'. Paper presented at A.S.H.A. Convention, Detroit, October 1973.

Stark, J. (1966). Performance of aphasic children on the ITPA. *Except. Child* **33**, 153–158.

Stark, J. (1967). A comparison of the performance of aphasic children on three sequencing tests. *J. Commun. Dis.* **1**, 31–34.

Tallal, P. (1975). Perceptual and linguistic factors in the language impairment of developmental dysphasics; an experimental investigation with the Token Test. *Cortex* **11**, 196–205.

Tallal, P. (1977). An Experimental Investigation of the Role of Auditory Temporal Processing in Normal and Disordered Language Development. *In* 'Acquisition and Breakdown of Language: Parallels and Divergencies' (A. Caramazza and E. Zuriff, eds). Johns Hopkins Press, Baltimore, Maryland.

Tallal, P. and Piercy, M. (1973a). Defects of non-verbal auditory perception in children with developmental dysphasia. *Nature* **241**, 468–499.

Tallal, P. and Piercy, M. (1973b). Developmental aphasia; Impaired rate of non-verbal processing as a function of sensory modality. *Neuropsychologia* **11**, 389–398.

Tallal, P. and Piercy, M. (1974). Developmental aphasia; Rate of auditory processing and selective impairment of consonant perception. *Neuropsychologia* **12**, 83–93.

Tallal, P. and Piercy, M. (1975). Developmental aphasia; The perception of brief vowels and extended stop consonants. *Neuropsychologia* **13**, 69–74.

Tallal, P., Stark, R. and Curtiss, B. (1976). The relation between speech perception impairment and speech production impairment in children with developmental dysphasia. *Brain and Language* **3**, 305–317.

Templin, M. C. (1957). 'Certain Language Skills in Children'. University of Minnesota Press, Minneapolis.

Whitaker, H. A. and Noll, J. D. (1972). Some linguistic parameters of the token test. *Neuropsychologia* **10**, 395–404.

Withrow, F. R. (1964). Immediate recall for aphasic, deaf, and normal children for visual forms presented simultaneously or sequentially. *ASHA* **6**, 386.

The Basis of Childhood Dysphasia: A Linguistic Approach

Richard F. Cromer

Introduction

There are basically two approaches to the study of any psychological behaviour. One consists in centring attention on the specific behaviour itself.
This approach leads to description, classification, and also to studies of a
correlational nature which attempt to interrelate various phenomena which
may be associated with the behaviour in question. Another approach, however, is to 'dig deeper' and to try to uncover the underlying processes (or
deficiencies) which lead to or produce the observed behaviour. Obviously
there must be an interaction between these two approaches. It is the
behavioural phenomenon that must, eventually, be understood or explained. But in order to know how to bring about changes in that behaviour, or to produce a remedial effect, one must come to an understanding of the basic processes that are affecting or causing that behaviour.
Moreover, quite different deficiencies may underlie the same or similar
observable phenomena – especially when those phenomena are abnormal
behaviour patterns.

There are dangers, however, in approaches that attempt to deal exclusively with the underlying processes. One of these stems from the fact
that the way in which underlying processes are conceived often reflects
one's assumptions about the structure of the behaviour itself. This becomes a danger because a particular conception becomes outmoded or
else reflects a contemporary misunderstanding of the structure of that
behaviour. A second problem is that one may lose sight of the behaviour
that is to be explained, and as a result hypotheses and theories put
forward are unable to account for that behaviour. A good example of this
was in the 1950s when the emphasis was put on stimuli, responses, frequencies, associational mechanisms and reinforcement principles as applied to language acquisition by the young child, with little awareness

that the actual language behaviour of young children differed considerably from the patterns that would be predicted on the basis of those processes. The study of disordered language is particularly vulnerable to these two problems. In the first place, one's understanding (or misunderstanding) of the nature of linguistic structure may greatly influence the search for the types of processes likely to be impaired and which therefore prevent language comprehension or production. Secondly, the hypothesised process impairments must be able to account for the kinds of disordered language actually observed. In the course of the first part of this chapter, the author will put forward the possibility that some of the recent work on the processing difficulties underlying childhood dysphasia may have been influenced by the shortcomings outlined above.

In an early paper, Lashley (1951) discussed the problem of serial order in behaviour. He pointed out the difficulties inherent in associative chain explanations of certain sequences of actions, for example rhythmic activity, typing, speech, and, most important for our purposes, grammatical structure. Lashley claimed that such sequences cannot be explained in terms of the successions of stimuli. Rather, underlying these overtly expressed sequences are a number of integrative processes which can only be inferred from the final results of their activity. This constitutes what Lashley called 'the essential problem of serial order', namely, the existence of generalised schemata which determine the sequence of specific actions. In line with this view Lashley, when looking specifically at language, claimed that any theory that describes grammatical form as due merely to the associative linkage of the words in the sentence overlooks its essential structure. This is also one of the main points made by recent linguistic theory (see Chomsky's 1959 criticism of Skinner's model of language acquisition). Miller and Chomsky (1963) have argued strongly against the theory which explains acquisition of linguistic structure in terms of sequential links. They demonstrated that any theory of language acquisition based on the sequence of words (Skinner, 1957) or even on the possible sequences of grammatical categories (Jenkins and Palermo, 1964) would be mathematically impossible for the child to learn. For example, in the relatively long sentence, 'The people who called and wanted to rent your house when you go away next year are from California', the listener detects a dependency between the 2nd word (people) and the 17th word (are) – a string of 15 sequential dependencies. The reader can easily demonstrate this to himself by substituting the word 'person' for 'people' or, alternatively, substituting 'is' for 'are', for this will produce a sentence which is unlikely to be uttered (or written) or which would jar the listener or reader if it were. Based on certain assumptions concerning the average number of categories in a given sentence, Miller and Chomsky estimated (conservatively) that the listener, in order to have detected this dependency, would have had to learn 10^9 different possible transitions between sequential grammatical categories in – as they put it – a childhood lasting only 10^8 seconds. It can similarly be demonstrated that attempts merely to modify sequential theories by notions such as context generalisation or by adding rules which allow one to insert or embed certain strings of linguistic elements within other strings are also inadequate. In any case, the idea of the ability to embed some structures within others implies the existence of that same underlying planning or integrative capacity which Lashley claimed to be necessary in order to explain externally observed sequences.

Despite this significantly different conception of language structure, the predominant emphasis in research on disordered language has been based on a sequential view of language units. In other words, the earlier assumption that language is a sequential ordering of elements has led to a great deal of research into temporal ordering difficulties in individuals with linguistic impairments. In view of the more recent assumption of the hierarchical nature of linguistic structure, it may be that the importance attributed to the processing of temporal order is misconceived. The results of a linguistic analysis of the written productions of some dsyphasic children, discussed later in this chapter, tentatively support the view that the difficulty with language in these children stems from an inability to deal with hierarchically ordered relationships of the type inherent in the structure of language. But before discussing that research it is useful to review some of the hypotheses advanced to account for language difficulties in dysphasic children.

Some Theories of Childhood Dysphasia

Dysphasia is generally defined as the disturbance or the loss of ability to comprehend, elaborate, or express language concepts. In adults this may take a variety of forms which have been classified in various manners, for example on the primary type of dysfunction (i.e. whether receptive or expressive), or else in terms of the nature of the language disturbance (i.e. whether the patient is agrammatical, anomic, etc.). Dysphasia in childhood, although it can sometimes be classified in similar ways, may in fact be very different in nature. In adult dysphasia, a previously functioning linguistic system has been impaired, whereas in developmental or even in early acquired dysphasia the child has been prevented from the initial acquisition of a complete language system. The underlying dysfunction in dysphasic children may furthermore be quite different from the impaired processes studied in the various types of adult dysphasia, although studies on adults may provide some interesting clues as to the nature of the dysfunction in children. There is also the additional problem that the basic defect may differ from one child to another, and this has led some researchers either to despair or to redefine childhood dysphasia to fit the purposes of their study. However, using certain criteria of exclusion, it is possible to obtain small numbers of subjects showing the same underlying difficulties, thus providing a homogeneous group. Griffiths (1972) provided a working definition of the condition when she described 'developmental aphasia' as being a failure of the normal growth of language function when deafness, mental deficiency, motor disability, or severe personality disorder can be excluded. Several researchers have noted an inattention and an inconsistency of response to sound (Benton, 1964; Eisenson, 1968; Lea, 1970; Petrie, 1975; Schuell in Millikan and Darley, 1967), although it is unclear whether this is a contributory cause or an effect of the language disability. The main theories put forward to account for the lack of language in dysphasic children are as follows: (a) a specific defect of auditory perception, (b) an impairment of the auditory storage system, (c) impairment of rhythmic ability, (d) a defect in sequencing and temporal ordering abilities, and (e) a specific, linguistic system impairment. These theories are briefly reviewed before presenting research findings which have shown that the linguistic structure of dysphasic (and deaf) children does not lend support to the theories so far proposed, the underlying difficulty in dysphasic children may lie in an impairment of a hierarchical structuring ability.

AUDITORY IMPERCEPTION

Word deafness or congenital auditory imperception implies that in spite of intact peripheral hearing mechanisms auditory speech cannot be processed by the central nervous system (see Worster-Drought and Allen, 1929). It is not easy to assess the auditory abilities of aphasic children. In addition to the inconsistency of response to sound, it is often noted that these children show no orienting reflex to sounds, even non-speech stimuli. Mark and Hardy (1958) studied 36 language handicapped children with auditory imperception (median age, $6\frac{1}{2}$ years) who had orienting reflex disturbances. These children failed to respond to newly introduced sounds and to sounds which elicit orienting responses in normal children. Psychogalvanic skin response audiometry established that the failure to respond to sound stimuli was not attributable to a peripheral hearing disorder. What, then, is the cause of their orienting reflex disturbance? Mark and Hardy collected evidence to show that a significant number of these children did possess, in infancy, an orienting reflex to sound. The evidence was derived from the study of the age at which the first symptom occurred – i.e. the earliest age at which the informants (usually the parents) 'had the slightest cloud of suspicion that anything at all was wrong with the child' – and the character of the alerting symptom (whether speech or response to sound). In addition, anecdotal evidence of early responses to sound was collected. Especially in cases when the first symptoms occurred late, there were also detailed reports of startle responses, orienting reflexes and readiness-to-listen behaviour patterns. In some cases there was even evidence of early sound imitation and speech, and in a very few cases expletive or interjectional speech in children who were later on considered totally non-speaking. Mark and Hardy attempted to account for the lack of orienting reflexes to sound at later ages by hypothesising that some cerebral damage or faulty development interfered in the establishment of the links between sounds and meaning. They argued that the child disregards sound later because the impressions from this sense modality remain unreinforced.

There are some problems with this interpretation. An inspection of the table in the Mark and Hardy paper reveals that in 23 of the 36 children the alerting symptom was a hearing symptom. But eleven of these were under 1 year of age, and six of these were less than 6 months old. It is somewhat difficult to see in what way a linkage between sound and meaning could be impaired at these very young ages to the extent of producing an apparent 'hearing' disturbance. More crucially, some experiments have shown that dysphasic children are not impaired in their ability to attach meaning to particular sounds (see, e.g. Barna, 1975, to be discussed in a later section). Rather than a link between sound and meaning, other researchers have argued that the basic impairment lies in the perception of speech sounds.

It may be that one major defect in dysphasic children is not the perception of sounds *per se*, but the perception of sounds in context. It is known, for example, that the perception of vowels is greatly dependent on context (Fry *et al.*, 1962). Eisenson (1968) has suggested that dysphasic children may suffer from an inability to generalise sounds into phonetic contexts. That is, they can discriminate phonemes, when presented in isolation but not when they are incorporated into phonetic contexts. He conjectured that this resulted from a narrow and premature rigidity of the speech categories of the dysphasic children. In an experimental study, McReynolds (1966) found that dysphasic children between the ages of four and eight years performed as well as normal children when discriminating isolated speech sounds, but did significantly worse when the same speech sounds were embedded in a phonetic context. McReynolds offered a number of possible explanations for this finding. But she seems to favour the above mentioned interpretation of Mark and Hardy, that is, a lack of reinforcement for auditory perceptual responses which has led to an inhibition in the response to auditory signals, especially in language-like tasks, in which the dysphasic child may have experienced constant failure. Thus the inhibitions for language-like signals are stronger and more habitual than they are for auditory signals which do not resemble language. Again, there are several problems with this interpretation. For example, why have these children been unrewarded for language behaviour in the past? If such poor reinforcement contingencies for language have led to the lack of auditory response, especially for language-like signals, then this lack of auditory response cannot be responsible for the poor language abilities in the first place. But more importantly, there is no proof that language development in normal children is based on especially good reinforcement contingencies.

McReynolds offers several other alternative explanations for her results. For example, she thinks that dysphasic children suffer from an inability to deal with more than one perceptual skill at a time. In the sounds-in-context task, the child must not only discriminate the sounds, but retain and sequence them, and the simultaneous use of these skills may be beyond the child's capabilities. On the other hand, it is possible that the impairment may be merely in the ability to sequence the sounds. Theories of these types will be discussed in later sections.

Rosenthal (1972) has suggested several possibilities to explain the performance of dysphasic children on auditory processing tasks (Rosenthal and Eisenson, 1970; Rosenthal, 1971). One of his theories postulates a basic auditory perceptual dysfunction. Rosenthal (1971) conducted an experiment designed to study the relationship between intensity of an auditory signal and its duration. He claimed that in normal subjects, at near threshold levels, the auditory system seems to summate or integrate the moment-to-moment energy into continuous signals. Consequently, if the duration of a signal is decreased, greater signal intensity would be required for detection. Since other experiments, however, appear to have demonstrated that dysphasic children are put at a severe disadvantage when temporal constraints are placed on auditory processing, Rosenthal hypothesised that signal intensities would have to be increased abnormally for this group in order to maintain normal detectability. The results were, in fact, somewhat equivocal. Only half of the dysphasic subjects showed a significant abnormal relationship between signal duration and detection thresholds. Nevertheless, as a group, the dysphasic subjects did require substantially greater increases in signal intensity than did the normal subjects. But there were other problems. These differences were only found at the shortest signal durations. Moreover, while the data at a 1000 Hz frequency supported Rosenthal's hypothesis, no reliable differences were found between dysphasic and normal subjects at a higher, 4000 Hz, frequency signal. He attempted to explain this in terms of a complex theory based on a notion of 'critical bands'. Basically, this theory holds that the ear does not respond to sounds outside particular frequency ranges (the critical band). The critical band for certain frequencies is thought to widen at short signal durations. Rosenthal suggests that in dysphasic children this widening of the critical band does not occur to the same extent as in normal children. Rosenthal raises the question of whether such critical bands are to be viewed as a fixed physical property, for example of the cochlear or other mechanism, or whether they are a function of some kind of internal filtering which is subject to cognitive control. In either case the possible cause of the child's lack of language ability may stem from a type of auditory imperception, but one which would not necessarily be limited to speech-like sounds.

IMPAIRMENT OF THE AUDITORY STORAGE SYSTEM

One explanation by McReynolds (1966) for the inability of dysphasic children to deal with sounds in context was mentioned earlier. It was claimed that in order to carry out such a task, the child had to make simultaneous use of more than one perceptual skill – for example, not only to discriminate sounds but to retain and sequence them. This view is compatible with theories which seek to explain the basic difficulty of dysphasic children as a limitation of auditory storage ability. While a number of experimental investigations have studied various aspects of auditory imperception, very little specific work has been done on this second type of theory. Eisenson (1968) speculated that the dysphasic child's storage system for speech signals may be defective. That is, immediate recall of signals measured by matching procedures may be adequate, but the storage of such signals may be defective.

There are some experiments concerned with sequencing disabilities in dysphasic children, the results of which, on the basis of the procedures used, could be interpreted as showing a memory storage problem. Stark et al. (1967) studied eight dysphasic children (mean age 8 years 3 months) and eight normal controls (mean age 5 years 3 months) on a task which involved depressing three keys with pictures on them, in the same order as the items were auditorally presented by the experimenter. Three of the dysphasics did well on the task but five did not. Of the errors made by these five children, 76 per cent occurred on the item in first position, whilst in the normal children and the other three dysphasics only 40 per cent of errors were on the first position. Furthermore, verbal stress put on the first item improved the scores of the five dysphasics, but did not help the normal children. Stark et al. (1967) concluded that the results showed that dysphasics have impaired auditory memory for sequences. The difficulty was mainly related to the forgetting of the first item in the sequence, but when the first item was stressed, recall of the entire sequence was enhanced. Although Stark *et al.* (1967) saw the inability primarily in terms of sequencing difficulty, it could be argued that what this experiment really shows is an impaired memory function in five of the eight dysphasic children.

Poppen *et al.* (1969), in a later set of experiments, studied visual sequencing by a similar technique. In one experiment, nine dysphasic children (mean age 9 years 3 months) and nine normal children (mean age 8 years 8 months), viewed pictures on three frosted panels. The task was to press the keys in the order they had flashed. The results will be discussed in more detail in the section on sequencing, but here it is relevant to note that when a delay (ranging from 2 to 17 seconds) was introduced between presentation and response the number of errors increased significantly; however, the delay had a greater effect on the dysphasic than on the normal children. Reading from the graph presented in their paper, it appears that the errors of the dysphasic group were about 25 per cent with a 2 second delay, but increased to 40 per cent with a 17 second delay. By contrast, the errors by the normal children increased from about 8 per cent (with a 2 second interval) to about 12 per cent (at a 17 second interval). Although Poppen *et al.* (1969) were mainly concerned with a sequencing explanation, they suggested that memory and attention may be basic to that ability.

Rosenthal (1972) was also concerned, in some of his experiments, with sequencing disabilities, specifically in the auditory modality; but his results are also compatible with a theory of an auditory storage impairment. In a study of temporal order effects Rosenthal and Eisenson (1970) presented short speech sounds, either singly or in pairs, to dysphasic and normal children. When the sounds occurred in pairs, the subject's task was to order them temporally, and the time taken to do this was compared with their performance on non-speech sounds which were similarly contrasting. The results showed that the dysphasic as well as the normal children could learn and later identify with a high degree of accuracy the stimuli which were presented singly. When those stimuli were paired in close temporal proximity, however, and the children had to report the order of their occurrence, performance by the dysphasic children broke down. Rosenthal and Eisenson take this as evidence that the nature of the auditory processing defect in dysphasic children is primarily one of short-term auditory storage. That is, the auditory trace, which can be identified singly, is not retained long enough to allow a perceptual analysis of temporal order; thus their interpretation of the difficulty of temporal ordering is that it results from an auditory storage deficit. Not all theories of sequencing disability agree with this, and many would emphasise that the temporal order dysfunction itself is the primary disability. It should be pointed out that these different theories will lead to different predictions.

A theory of auditory memory impairment would appear to predict greater difficulty with increasing numbers of auditory items, whereas temporal ordering disabilities, which will be discussed in a later section, should affect even the shortest auditory strings.

IMPAIRMENT OF RHYTHMIC ABILITY

Clinical observations often suggest that certain types of adult dysphasic patients (e.g. those diagnosed as suffering from conduction aphasia), have difficulty reproducing non-verbal rhythmic sequences (Tzortzis and Albert, 1974). One of the most common observations by those who work closely with dysphasic children is that these children lack the ability to appreciate or deal with rhythm. Griffiths (1972) reported that dysphasic children show 'an almost uniformly poor sense of rhythm' in such lessons and activities as music and movement, dancing, and singing. She studied 24 dysphasic children, six of whom were considered to be receptive dysphasics, while the remaining 18 were classified as expressive dysphasics. These children ranged in age from 6 years 9 months to 9 years 10 months (mean 7 years 11 months), and their IQs from 70 to 128 (mean 98) on the Performance or Full Scale of the WISC. They were compared with 40 normal children on a number of tasks involving the sequencing of digits, the comprehension and repetition of sentences, and the repetition of non-verbal rhythms. This last task required the child to repeat a rhythm on a tambourine, immediately after the experimenter. There were four rhythm tests, each consisting of ten items arranged in increasing order of complexity. The results showed that while the dysphasic children were less successful on all of the tasks than the normal children, the task which most sharply differentiated the groups was the rhythm repetition task. The errors made by normal children on the rhythms tended to be very minor. But Griffiths reports that, when the dysphasic children attempted to copy the rhythms, their productions often showed no apparent relationship to the rhythmic pattern presented, and gave the impression that some of their 'successes' were a matter of chance.

When certain disabilities are observed in a group, one must always question whether those disabilities are the cause or merely the effect of the basic condition by which the group is defined. In an early paper, Rosenstein (1957) assumed that the absence of hearing should have a significant effect on the ability to perceive rhythmic patterns, even if these rhythms are presented in a non-auditory modality. He used 30 pairs of rhythmic patterns presented tactually and compared matched groups of normal, blind, deaf, and dysphasic children. The task was to render a judgement of 'same' or 'different' to the second of two vibratory rhythms delivered to the right index fingertip. Contrary to prediction, the blind group performed best, with the deaf, dysphasics, and normals performing about equally and more poorly than the blind. Rosenstein felt, however, that there was some support for his hypothesis, since with practice the two normally hearing groups (the blind and the normals) improved their performance slightly, while the two groups who suffered from an auditory impairment (the deaf and the dysphasics) did not. Rosenstein concluded that auditory experience perhaps plays some role in the *improvement* of rhythmic discrimination, but he admits that his results do not show that auditory experience contributed to superior *initial* rhythmic discrimination.

Kracke (1975) starts with a different assumption, based on observations of deaf and of dysphasic children. She claims that these children display many behavioural similarities including 'normal play activities, good inter-personal relationships, efficient non-verbal communication between the children, not much verbal interaction, (and) little reaction to sound in-cluding their own names'. There is, however, one very noticeable differ-ence. Deaf children are observed to enjoy rhythmic activities such as clapping, dancing, and using percussion instruments. Dysphasic children, by contrast, cannot clap or beat rhythms which they hear and often are out of step with each other's movements. Kracke tested this observed difference experimentally; the aim of the study was also to ascertain whether the rhythmic disability is specific to the auditory modality or whether it transcends it. After a series of warm-up tasks to get the children to render same and different judgements to various pairs of stimuli, Kracke presented rhythmic patterns consisting of three stimuli, repeated three times to make up a rhythmic sequence. This was compared to a subsequent rhythmic sequence for a 'same' or 'different' judgement. Twelve comparisons were made on auditory rhythms, and twelve on rhythms which were applied to the child's fingertips by a vibrating disc. Twelve children were tested in each of the three groups (i.e. receptive dysphasic, profoundly deaf, and normal children) matched for sex, age (8 years 4 months to 15 years 3 months), and non-verbal intelligence. The auditory rhythms were presented at levels of high intensity for the deaf children, and only children who could hear the experimental tones were included in the experiment. The results showed that, regardless of modality, the hearing and the profoundly deaf performed similarly, with the average number of correct responses of the two groups on the two tasks between 10·3 and 11·6 out of 12 rhythmic sequences. By contrast, the dysphasic children performed significantly worse, the group average of correct responses being only 6·6 for rhythms presented auditorally, and 5·8, for the vibrotactile rhythms. Thus, it seems clear that the deaf do not suffer a deficit in rhythmic ability, but dsyphasic children do. Kracke claims that some underlying process apparently fails in dysphasic chil-dren, a process which enables unimpaired subjects 'to learn to recognise lawful relationships in temporal gestalts'. If this process is impaired, it may well have an important effect on sentence perception. These results, with a slight change of emphasis on the interpretation of what this disability may be, will be discussed in the final part of this chapter when several findings are brought together. Furthermore, it should be noted that Kracke's results suggest that the rhythmic disability is not limited to the auditory modality, but is of a nature that transcends other sense modalities.

The findings briefly reviewed here indicate that even profoundly deaf children do not suffer impairment of rhythmic ability. Rosenstein's results also support this conclusion, although in fact he started with the opposite assumption. What remains puzzling is the fact that, in his experiment, the dysphasic children were not especially impaired on rhythms when compared to the deaf and normal groups, despite the common observation concerning their poor performance on such tasks.

SEQUENCING AND TEMPORAL ORDER DEFICITS

There is another area of study where there is some question as to whether the hypothesised deficit is limited to the auditory modality or whether it is more general in nature – sequencing and temporal order deficits. Problems of temporal disorientation and temporal ordering in certain types of brain damaged patients have been discussed for some time (e.g. Hughlings-Jackson, 1888; Critchley, 1953). Hirsh (1959) emphasised the importance of a central temporal sequencing ability for making sense of auditory input and language. Monsees (1961) speculated that the basic disability in dysphasic children was a central disorder involving the perception of temporal sequence. The most commonly cited early experimental work on the impairment of such abilities in dysphasic patients, however, was that by Efron (1963). He found that in adult dysphasics, the ability to say which of two sounds occurred first was seriously impaired unless the two stimuli were separated by a gap of as much as 575 ms. This was contrasted with the fact that in normal speech sound segments occur approximately every 80 ms. It was suggested, therefore, that dysphasic patients are unable to process normal speech because they cannot sort out the temporal order of the phonemes. That such sequencing may be important at the phoneme level is also supported by a study made by Sheehan et al. (1973). They found that the comprehension of some adult dysphasics was aided by the insertion of silent intervals between phonemes, but not by the insertion of silence between words. Efron (1963), however, commented on the difficulties that exist in this simplistic interpretation of the findings. For example, the dysphasic adults who showed the poorest performances on his temporal ordering task were patients with expressive dysphasia,

while those with receptive difficulties had little trouble with auditory
sequencing. That is, the expressive dysphasics who needed so large an
intervening gap between auditory stimuli in order to sequence them
correctly, nevertheless understood normal speech, even though this
comes at the rate of one phoneme per 80 ms. Efron admits that these
findings are puzzling, and as he later put it in Millikan and Darley (1967)
there is no significant correlation between the severity of the dysphasia
and the degree of difficulty these patients have with sequencing. Some
patients who understand speech reasonably well are very poor on a
sequencing task. Others, who are profoundly dysphasic, score near normal
results on sequencing. Further studies have turned up similar conflicting
findings. Malone (1967) examined the relationship between the ability of
dysphasics to resolve the temporal order of pure tones differing in frequency, and to identify sentences played at rapid speeds. No relationship
was found between these two tasks (r = 0·08). Indeed, subjects were able
to identify speech even when its mean rate of presentation exceeded their
rate for ordering two tones by a ratio of more than two to one. Rees
(1973), relying on evidence of this type, criticises theories of dysphasia
based on auditory processing difficulties. She cites Day's (1970) hypothesis
that there are at least two different levels of temporal order perception
– a non-linguistic and a higher, more potent, linguistic level. Theories
based on auditory processing of discrete phonemes or speech sound segments will not be able to explain the perception of connected speech.
Experiments like those of Bever *et al.* (1969), in which it was shown that
the processing of sentences is carried out on the basis of major clause constituents, are taken as evidence that there is no basis for the assumption
that the comprehension of heard speech depends on a more fundamental
ability to analyse utterances into an ordered set of phoneme strings.

Perhaps these linguistic experiments provide a clue to the partial
solution of Efron's puzzle. The adult expressive dysphasics who can
comprehend speech yet need a large separation of two signals to make a
correct judgement of temporal order may, in some sense, be relying on
formerly learned language patterns in order to process sentences. They
are, after all, people who prior to their illness possessed a normal language
system, and having once known a linguistic system they can make use of
different processing mechanisms, such as Day's (1970) higher order
linguistic processing, to understand speech even when its rate exceeds
that necessary to order temporally non-linguistic stimuli. By contrast, a
temporal order disability in children could prevent them from acquiring
a full linguistic system in the first place, and could conceivably be the
cause of their dysphasia.

Lowe and Campbell (1965) studied auditory temporal processes in a
group of children classified as 'aphasoid'. Eight such children, aged 7 to

14 years, were compared with a group of matched normal-speaking children. Two types of temporal tasks were studied: 'succession' tasks to measure the amount of time required by a subject in order for him to hear two auditory events as separate events, and 'temporal ordering' tasks to measure the slightly greater amount of time which is needed for the subject to be able to state which of the two auditory events occurred first. In succession tasks, the aphasoid children needed, on average, 35·8 ms compared to the normal average of 18·5 ms. This difference, however, did not reach statistical significance. On the temporal ordering task, the aphasoid children required 357 ms as compared to only 36·1 ms by normal children. This very large difference was highly significant. Furthermore, since the average of 357 ms required by the aphasoid children is far above the rate of normal speech (80 ms per phoneme), Lowe and Campbell concluded that temporal order malfunction may be the major factor in the language difficulties in these children.

Tallal and Piercy (1973a, b, 1974, 1975) have conducted a series of studies on temporal order processing by dysphasic children. They have found that when the rate of presentation of two stimuli is too great, the child is not able to ascertain their order of occurrence. But Tallal and Piercy do not conclude that the impairment is one of sequencing inability as such. Rather, they believe that the basic inability is an impairment in the rate of auditory processing, to which a sequencing difficulty is secondary. That is, for developmental dysphasics, the time available for auditory processing is critical for adequate performance. Their performance improves when the rate of presentation of stimuli is reduced, as was done in these experiments either by increasing the durations of the stimuli or by increasing the interval between them (cf. Sheehan et al., 1973). Tallal and Piercy also note, however, that the dysphasic children were impaired on all auditory serial memory tasks even when the durations and the interstimulus-intervals were maximal. It is therefore necessary to postulate additional deficits, such as a specific defect of auditory memory, or the need by these children for disproportionately more time to process more elements (Tallal and Piercy, 1973b).

In spite of the need for additional explanations, Tallal and Piercy nevertheless emphasise the importance of the lowered speed of processing in the auditory modality shown by these children. It may, indeed, have the effect of causing difficulty in discriminating speech sounds. In a recent experiment (1974), Tallal and Piercy found that dysphasic children have difficulty in discriminating between stop consonants which have rapidly changing spectrums provided by the 2nd and 3rd formant transitions, which in fact are of relatively short duration (50 ms). By contrast, they show no difficulty in discriminating vowels which have steady-state frequencies of the first three formants which remain constant over the entire length of the stimulus (approximately 250 ms). That is, Tallal and Piercy found that dysphasic children performed as well as matched non-dysphasic normal children on the vowels, but their performance was significantly worse on the stop consonants. Indeed, only 5 of the 12 dysphasic children were even able to make the initial discrimination between two stop consonants. It could be, of course, that dysphasic children suffer from an inability to process transitional stimuli, regardless of their duration, and that this is why they performed adequately on the vowels but not on the consonants. To test this, Tallal and Piercy (1975) used a new set of stimuli including specially synthesised vowel-vowel syllables in which the discriminable acoustic information occurred only within the first 43 ms of the stimuli. These differ from the consonant-vowel syllables, which also contain the discriminable information in the first 43 ms, in that the information in the former is of a steady-state character, while that in the latter is of a transitional nature. In conjunction with this they tested consonant-vowel stimuli but modified these so that the initial transitional period of each stimulus was increased from 43 ms to 95 ms although they were still of a transitional nature. The results showed that the dysphasic children were impaired when the discriminable components of the two stimuli were brief (43 ms) but unimpaired when these components were longer (95 ms), regardless of whether or not they were transitional in nature. Thus, the impairment in dysphasic children's discrimination of consonants is due to the brief duration of the discriminable components. Tallal and Piercy (1975) conclude that the language defect in dysphasic children is not specifically linguistic but is secondary to an impairment in the ability to process rapidly occurring auditory information. Their argument seems to be that this impaired processing ability underlies the sequencing difficulties which they have observed in the auditory modality. In other words, sequencing difficulties and the language deficits thought to be associated with them are seen as the effects of this auditory processing impairment.

There are some grounds for raising doubts, not only about this conclusion, but about the other theories which, by contrast, attach a central causative role to sequencing disabilities. Firstly, is the defect in these children specifically auditory as Tallal and Piercy claim it is? Secondly, when considering theories of sequencing disabilities in dysphasic children, are such disabilities a primary cause of the dysphasia, as most of these theories seem to hold, or are they merely an effect? Thirdly, do any of these theories really explain the difficulties which are observed in dysphasic children? We can examine these three questions in turn.

Is the sequencing deficit specifically auditory? A number of researchers have suggested that dysphasic children suffer from a general sequencing disability which is not limited to the auditory modality. Withrow (1964) studied immediate memory for sequentially presented visual stimuli in dysphasic, deaf, and normally-hearing children. He reported that both the deaf and the dysphasic children performed significantly worse than the normal children. Poppen *et al.* (1969), in an experiment mentioned earlier, asked six dysphasic children (aged 5 years 8 months to 9 years 3 months) to press three frosted panels in the same order they had seen them lighted. Although they performed better on this visual task than on auditory sequencing tasks, they still only achieved a 75 per cent success rate. In another part of their paper, these authors reported the correlations among several different sequencing tasks, which included both auditory and visual modalities, in the dysphasic and normal children groups. They felt that the high intercorrelations (Kendall's coefficient of concordance for five sequencing tasks being 0·716) lent support to the notion that there is a general sequencing ability and that dysphasic children are deficient in that ability.

The evidence for visual sequencing deficits in dysphasic children is not as strong as that for auditory sequencing deficits, and whereas in some experiments a trend towards impairment appears it does not quite reach significance. For example, Furth (1964) tested the ability to learn visual sequences in dysphasic, normal, and deaf children. The task consisted in learning to associate two-term sequences of shapes with a number. These nonsense shapes were presented sometimes simultaneously (thus requiring the learning of a left/right ordering) and sometimes successively. As these conditions did not differ in any of the three groups, the scores for both types of sequencing were combined. The overall task scores showed a great overlap among the groups, with the hearing children scoring the fewest errors (mean errors = 34·5) followed by the deaf with a score of 41·3. The dysphasic children scored the greatest number of errors (56·5). The mean number of errors by the deaf children did not differ significantly from either the normal or the dysphasic children, and the difference between the normals and the dysphasics was only significant at the 0·10 level. Furth points out, however, that the sequences consisted of only two elements and that all of the dysphasic children in his group had been receiving sequencing training for a number of years. These factors in fact may have precluded him from obtaining a clear-cut result in his experiment; however, a strong trend towards poorer sequencing ability in this visual task was shown by the dysphasic children. Stark (1967) tested 30 dysphasic children (aged 4 years 6 months to 8 years 2 months, mean IQ 76·8 on the Stanford-Binet), with three sequencing tasks. These three tests were the Knox Cube Tapping Task in which the subject must imitate the order of a series of taps which are graded in difficulty, and two sub-tests from the Illinois Test of Psycholinguistic Abilities (ITPA) (one auditory and one a visual sequencing task). Stark found that the dysphasic children scored significantly below their age level on all three tasks. On the other hand, Olson (1961) found no differences between deaf and dysphasic children on the same two sub-tests of the ITPA. Since neither of these experiments used normal control groups, it is difficult to interpret the results. In Olson's experiment, the deaf and dysphasics performed similarly; but it is not clear whether both groups performed average or below on the sequencing tasks. In Stark's study, dysphasic children performed below their age level on sequencing; but in his particular group a low score was not unexpected as their mean IQ was only 76·8 (although it is important to note that the mean was 95·9 on an adaptation of the non-verbal Leiter International Performance Scale).

Some other experiments, while not concerned with sequencing, have shown a possible involvement of some aspects of the visual cognitive function. Wilson et al. (1960) for example attempted to teach a group of dysphasic children to identify sounds. Their original hypothesis was that certain kinds of perceptual discrimination are difficult for dysphasic children. The stimuli they used consisted of sounds varying in two values (long and short) on two dimensions (duration and quality). Thus, the child had to learn four stimuli (a long tone, a short tone, a long noise, and a short noise) and to associate these with four randomly selected letters of the alphabet. Fourteen children with receptive dysphasia (mean age 8 years 1 month, mean IQ 114) were compared to thirteen non-dysphasic children (mean age 8 years 5 months, mean IQ 120). The group of non-dysphasic children was from the same clinic as the dysphasic group, and ten of these non-dysphasics suffered from hearing loss. The task was to point to the correct letter of the four, each mounted on a 7 in × 8 in card, in response to the particular sound. The criterion of learning was six consecutive correct responses, and training was discontinued if learning was not achieved in 80 trials. The results showed that the dysphasic children were not a homogeneous group. Thus, out of the fourteen, six never achieved criterion, while all thirteen non-dysphasic children achieved criterion with 50 trials. On the other hand, three dysphasic children with the best scores equalled the three best scores of the deaf children. An analysis of errors showed that dysphasic children generally made more errors for short stimuli and had more difficulty discriminating the quality of short sounds. While this may appear to support a hypothesis concerning the specific auditory nature of the deficit, further observations by Wilson et al. (1960) lead to a different conclusion. The dysphasic children who had been unable to learn the task were given post-training sessions. It was found that the task was made easier if only a single card was shown and the auditory stimulus repeated several times. With this kind of training, all the children were able to form the correct associations. There was also greater success when all the individual cards were visible; whilst when all four letters were on one card, only one child was successful. Wilson *et al.* (1960) conclude that the inability to learn shown in the main experiment most likely resulted from 'the complexity of the associative process' rather than from a deficit on the perceptual discrimination of the four acoustic stimuli. One could, of course, argue the opposite; the informal procedure in which the stimuli were repeated several times provided better opportunities to learn the auditory discrimination. But Wilson *et al.* (1960) present still further informal evidence. Two dysphasic and two non-dysphasic children were given a task of discriminating a tone and white noise of different duration. The results showed that all four children could correctly discriminate tone from noise on all trials even when the stimulus duration was reduced to 0·02 s. They could learn to say 'long tone', 'short tone', 'long noise', 'short noise' to the same stimuli used in the original experiment even after a single demonstration. Therefore, their failure could not originate from a difficulty in discriminating sounds. Indeed, repeating the original learning task still took one subject 37 trials. Wilson *et al.* (1960) conclude that the failure appears to be specific to the association between visually presented letters and auditory stimuli, and not because of any special difficulty of auditory discrimination.

Doehring (1960) carried out a visual task in groups of dysphasic, deaf, and normal hearing children, divided into two age ranges, 7 years 8 months to 9 years 7 months and 9 years 8 months to 11 years 7 months. The task was to draw an 'X' exactly where a spot of light, 5 mm in diameter, had been flashed. The experimental design included variations in exposure time (0·25 up to 3·5 s); variations in the time between presentation and response (1 s and 8 s); and he also studied the effect of interference and no interference with visual fixation conditions. Errors were evaluated by measuring the distance of the 'X' drawn by the children to the place where the light had actually flashed. Results showed that the dysphasic children performed significantly worse on this task than the normal or deaf children. The deaf were worse than the normal children, but not significantly so. There were significant effects of delay and of interference but these were almost identical for the three groups. There were significantly more errors made by the younger children than by the older children, and the older of the two dysphasic groups performed similarly to the younger of the two deaf and normal groups. Thus, in respect to accuracy on this task, dysphasic children might be supposed to be retarded by about two years. The delay of eight seconds before being allowed to respond did not disrupt dysphasic children any more than deaf or normal children, and so one could assume that these dysphasic children are not retarded in that aspect of visual memory. Doehring (1960) concludes that dysphasic children appear to be normal in the visual symbolic processes associated with delayed response, but they are retarded in the accuracy of their visual memory for spatial location.

Tzortzis and Albert (1974) studied sequencing behaviour in three adults with conduction dysphasia. Such patients are often said to be deficient in memory for the specific sequential order of items. Tzortzis and Albert set out to find whether this defect was specifically one of auditory-verbal short-term memory or whether it was a general deficit in memory for sequences. They administered a battery of 27 tests, among them repetition tests which varied both input (auditory or visual) and response (oral or pointing); matching tests in which strings of one to four letters, words, or numbers were followed by a similar or different sequence (requiring the subject to give a same/different judgement); tests of serial speech; and a rhythm test. The three patients with conduction dysphasia were com- pared with a patient recovering from Wernicke's dysphasia, and with one recovering from Broca's dysphasia; they also tested three normal subjects. The conduction dysphasics were found to have an impaired memory for sequences, and this was true whether the material was verbal or non-verbal, whether the modality of input was auditory or visual, and whether the response was oral or by pointing. It was observed that these dys-phasics could often produce all the items in a sequence correctly, but not the sequence itself. Tzortzis and Albert emphasise that the deficit could not have been purely auditory since these three dysphasics performed poorly even when the input was visual – although their performance was better than that for auditory stimuli. So the basic disorder in these patients with conduction dysphasia seems to lie in their inability to order elements in a sequence, even when they can remember the items that make up the sequence. It was also found that these same subjects had very poor scores on the rhythmic tapping task, and Tzortzis and Albert point out that this is consistent with the clinical observation that patients with conduction dysphasia have great difficulty in maintaining rhythms.

This report on adult dysphasics is included because it deals with the condition in which sequencing is considered the primary difficulty, and Tzortzis and Albert appear to have shown that a sequencing difficulty is not limited to the auditory system. This is contrary to the findings of Tallal and Piercy who claim to have shown that children with develop-mental dysphasia do not have difficulty with visual sequences. On an admittedly very different group of subjects, but in contrast to some of the other studies in children with developmental dysphasia (e.g. Furth, 1964; Poppen et al., 1969; Stark, 1967; and Withrow, 1964) Tallal and Piercy (1973b) claim that sequencing difficulty is found only in the auditory modality. They studied the performance of 12 dysphasic children (aged 6 years 9 months to 9 years 3 months) on two types of serial memory – one composed of two different tones and the other composed of two different lights (different shades of green). In this task, the child was trained to press a panel on the right for one tone (or light), and a panel on the left for the other. Serial patterns of three, four, and five elements were actually made up of only the two stimuli. In other tasks, in which only two-element patterns were used, the duration of the tone (or light) was varied as was the inter-stimulus interval. Both of these were kept constant in the longer serial memory task, although in one condition the duration of the stimuli was 75 ms and in the other 250 ms. Compared to twelve normal children matched for age, sex, and non-verbal intelligence, the dysphasics performed significantly worse on the 75 ms tones for three, four, and five element patterns. Whereas all of the normal children reached criterion (p < 0·001, binomial test) for all lengths, only two of twelve dysphasics reached criterion for strings of three elements, and only one of twelve on any longer pattern. When the tones were of 250 ms duration, however, the dysphasic children improved; ten of the twelve reached criterion on three-element patterns. But with four- and five-element patterns, only seven and two respectively reached criterion, and this was significantly worse than the normal children who all reached criterion on all the patterns. On the perceptual tasks (two elements) dysphasic subjects were significantly impaired both when the inter-stimulus intervals and the durations of the tones were decreased. By contrast, when visual stimuli were used no difference appeared between the dysphasic and normal children on any task, whether perceptual or serial memory.

It is not clear why some experiments show deficits of visual sequencing in dysphasic children whilst others do not. The argument is important because, if visual sequencing is disturbed, theories of developmental dysphasia which place the underlying cause in an auditory deficit will, at the very least, have to be elaborated to explain such visual defects. Tallal and Piercy (1973b), in fact, tentatively do just that. They point out that in the experiments in which some visual deficit has been observed, the visual sequences were presented spatially, whereas their own presentations were in fact temporal sequences presented in one location. Another difference was that Tallal and Piercy's procedure allowed the child to respond as soon as the stimuli were completed, whereas in some of the other experiments there was a delay before the children were allowed to respond. Tallal and Piercy speculate that these factors may have made some verbal mediation necessary, thus placing the dysphasic children at a disadvantage on the visual tasks. Precisely why verbal mediation would be made necessary was not made clear in their discussion, and in this respect it is important to note that rats and pigeons are capable of delayed responses. It is true that the tasks in the various experiments have been different, and one could argue, for example, that Tallal and Piercy's serial memory task is not a sequencing or temporal order task at all. Indeed,

Tallal and Piercy carefully avoid using the term 'sequencing' for their test, as it consisted of ordering serially two elements into longer strings. The other experimenters used either pictures, nonsense shapes, or spatial positions, with each element in the sequence being different from all others. Given the wide differences that exist in the various experimental designs, the debate over whether developmentally dysphasic children suffer from a broad sequencing defect or from a specifically auditory one is likely to continue. But there are other reasons for asking whether sequencing deficits of any type are in fact the cause of developmental dysphasia.

Is the sequencing disability a primary cause of the dysphasia? Most of the work on sequencing and temporal order difficulties assumes that a dysfunction in this area is responsible for the child being unable to comprehend language. The early findings of Efron (1963) on dysphasic adults and of Lowe and Campbell (1965) on 'aphasoid' children, for example, were taken as evidence that the auditory input of phonemes was too rapid for the individual to be able to sort out the order of occurrence; language would sound all jumbled up. But although a number of the above mentioned experiments seem to support the conclusion that auditory sequencing is disturbed in dysphasic children (whether as a primary dysfunction or as the result of a deficit in the rate of auditory processing) it is open to question whether this disability is really the *cause* of the dysphasic condition.

An experiment by Furth (1964), cited earlier, showed that dysphasic children responded poorly in a sequencing task, but their scores, while much lower than those of the normal and deaf groups, did not reach statistical significance. Furth speculated that one possible reason for this was that the dysphasic children had been receiving sequencing training in a special school for a number of years. Stark (1967) uses the same argument when discussing both the results of Furth and those of Olson (1961) who had found no differences between deaf and dysphasic children. Stark argues that the dysphasic children who participated in both experiments had received a number of years of training in sequence learning. But such an argument surely undermines the claimed causal nature of this disability. If a child is capable of being successfully trained in sequence learning, then this ability cannot be basically impaired. Furthermore, there is no evidence that successful sequence training alleviated their dysphasia.

It may be noted that dysphasic children are often compared not only with normal, but with deaf children in sequencing experiments. One of the reasons for this is that the deaf too are often thought to be deficient in temporal sequencing abilities. It should also be noted however, that when experimentation has shown the deaf to be poorer than normal children in sequencing, no one supposes their inability to sequence to be a *cause* of the deafness! The experiments with dysphasic children are of an identical logical status, but this does not appear to prevent some theorists from adopting the position that a sequencing disability is the cause of the dysphasia. In fact the direction of causation may be reversed; it may be that lack of experience with the auditory information of language, in these children, may result in their seldom relying on temporal order to encode or understand the world. O'Connor and Hermelin have been conducting a number of interesting experiments on deaf children and their ability to deal with temporally ordered phenomena. In one experiment (Hermelin and O'Connor, 1973), they used an ingenious technique in which various short strings of numbers were presented in a manner compatible with both spatial (left-to-right) and with temporal (first-to-last) coding. The apparatus consisted of three small windows arranged horizontally, and a fourth window, on its own, below them. In one situation three numbers appeared in the upper windows one after the other, but in such a way as not to occur in a left-to-right order. For example, if three numbers occurred in the temporal order 3, 9, 7, the spatial order might have 7 in the left-hand window, 3 in the central window, and 9 in the right-hand window. Thus the temporal order 397 would have appeared spatially as 739. After a one-second pause, a recognition display was exposed in the window below. It showed the same numbers exposed one after another, and this recognition display could show the numbers as they had appeared in temporal order (397), spatial order (739), or else randomly (e.g. 973). In a second condition, the initial presentation was successive, in the lower window, and the recognition task was based on the subsequent three-window display. Again, the three-window display could be presented temporally (but not spatially), spatially (but not temporally) or randomly. In both conditions, the child's task was to judge whether the order of the two presentations was the same or different. Hermelin and O'Connor found that normal hearing children generally gave temporally ordered recognition responses. Indeed, only 3 out of 40 hearing children (7·5 per cent) recognised the left-to-right but not the first-to-last order of the digits. By contrast, 31 out of 57 deaf children (54·4 per cent) recognised the spatially ordered display but not the temporally ordered one. In other words, even when the spatial display element was eliminated, from either the initial input or from the recognition display, more than half of the deaf children failed to recognise the previously presented temporal sequence. Such results appear to show an inability by many deaf children to deal with temporally ordered information, and many researchers would have been satisfied with such a conclusion. O'Connor and Hermelin (1973a, b),

however, carried out additional experiments. In one of these (1973a), 20
hearing and 20 congenitally deaf children viewed sets of either 5 photographs of faces or 5 nonsense syllables presented in 5 windows. As in their
first experimental technique mentioned above, the sequential (temporal,
first-to-last) order of the items was incongruent with a spatial (left-to-right)
order. In another condition 40 deaf and 40 hearing children saw similar
items presented successively at the same location. In both conditions, the
task was the same. After viewing the material, the children were shown
two temporally adjacent members of the set of five, and they had to tell
the experimenter which one had come first. Thus, in this experiment, the
children were clearly instructed to retain only temporal order information.
The results showed that in general there were no differences between
the hearing and deaf children on this task. The deaf performed better on the
photographs than on the nonsense syllables, and their performance on the
photographs was better than that of the normal children. The normally
hearing children were better on the nonsense syllables than on the photographs, and showed better results on the nonsense syllables than did the
deaf children. What is significant here is that when the deaf are instructed
to retain only temporally ordered information, they are as efficient as
hearing children. In the experiments mentioned previously, most deaf
children, when given an option, 'preferred' to remember the left-to-right
rather than the first-to-last temporal order. But according to O'Connor and
Hermelin the later experiment shows that in deaf children this is an
elective strategy rather than an incapacity to appreciate temporal order.

In the deaf children, then, lack of auditory input does not prevent them
from being able to appreciate temporal order, but it makes these children
unlikely to use that mode of ordering. In children with developmental
dysphasia, a temporal order disability has been observed, but it remains
to be shown whether this is 'elective' or not. The notion that such a
disability 'causes' the dysphasia, however, should be subjected to greater
scrutiny than it has in the past. Indeed, if a temporal ordering disability
does underlie the dysphasic condition in these children, one would expect
it to affect language in a defined and predictable manner. But this also
appears not to be the case.

Does the sequencing disability explain the observed language difficulties? This
chapter began with the assertion that recent work on the processes
underlying childhood dysphasia was subject to difficulty in two areas. The
first of these concerned the common assumption that language is serially
structured, and it was suggested that this view has exerted an influence on
the underlying processes which are thought to be defective in dysphasic
children. This section is exploring the hypothesis that directly reflects
such an assumption that some sort of sequencing disability is the cause of

developmental dysphasia. The second problem was said to be the danger of losing sight of the behaviour which was to be explained. If a sequencing disability is responsible for childhood dysphasia, effects of this disability should be at least partly reflected in the language behaviour of these children. If individuals cannot process the incoming auditory signal rapidly enough to determine the relative ordering of the elements, language would presumably appear to be jumbled and disordered. As mentioned in an earlier section, however, Efron (1967) reported, from his work with adult dysphasics, that no relation could be found between the severity of the dysphasia and the degree of difficulty with sequencing. He had noticed that some patients who were profoundly dysphasic scored near normal results on sequencing tasks. More significantly, a number of patients whom he described as 'hopeless' on sequencing tasks could nevertheless understand speech reasonably well. Geschwind (1967) also reported that some adult dysphasic patients with good auditory comprehension were defective in temporal ordering abilities. Furthermore, there were some dysphasic patients with impaired comprehension who nevertheless showed the ability to repeat perfectly. Geschwind concluded that in these cases the disturbance could not possibly be due to a defect in auditory temporal ordering ability. In these patients, for example, the sounds had to be perceived in the correct order to make exact repetition possible. In developmental dysphasia there is also no evidence that speech sounds appear jumbled to the child, nor indeed are there reports that these children produce temporally displaced phonological elements when attempting to speak. Rosenthal (1972), whose research has been reviewed in the sections on auditory imperception and auditory storage, reports problems similar to those encountered in the adult dysphasic research. For example, he states that all of the older children who were subjects in his experiments possessed usable language in spite of the fact that most of them were found to have impaired auditory processing abilities. Although he suggests that such a disorder in dysphasic children may interfere with the establishment of a phonological base for language, he admits that the language systems of these children also show phonological, syntactic, and semantic deviations. One suggestion is that auditory dysfunction does not adequately account for developmental dysphasia. Similarly, the notion of impaired sequencing abilities does not appear to explain adequately the observed syntactic deviations in these children. For example, if the sequencing difficulty is conceived as purely auditory in nature and is at the level of the phoneme or stop consonant, one would expect dysphasic children to exhibit jumbled words, not jumbled grammar. Furthermore, if the problem is one of sequencing in the auditory modality alone, then one might expect dysphasic children to be able to acquire language easily by lip reading or to acquire written language through a visual medium. As will be pointed out this does not appear to be the case and the errors made in language behaviour in other modalities are not, in the main, errors attributable to ordering difficulties which a broader sequencing-impairment theory might predict. Psychologists often seem peculiarly reluctant to explore the hypothesis which most directly reflects dysphasic language difficulties – that the disorder might be due to a specific linguistic system impairment which transcends the particular modality of linguistic input.

SPECIFIC LINGUISTIC SYSTEM IMPAIRMENT

One theoretical position which has not been explored adequately is that the dysphasic child suffers from some kind of basic linguistic impairment. According to this hypothesis, the child is unable to process those basic grammatical relations similar to the type suggested to exist as part of some kind of 'language acquisition device'. Chomsky (1965) has speculated that the ability to perceive and acquire certain linguistic relations is innate in the child. This speculation is based on a number of observations including the rapidity with which children in all cultures and subcultures acquire language, with or without emphasis on language tuition; the similar ages, worldwide, at which children become proficient in their various native languages; and the hypothesis that there are broad similarities, for all languages, in the children's use of early linguistic productions, even when these do not match in many instances the adult model. From the psychologist's point of view, it is not easy to specify what such a language acquisition device might contain, and it is therefore difficult to design experiments or make observations which would elucidate its content or structure. It would seem that there are several possibilities as to the nature of this species-specific, language-directed behaviour. One could argue, for example, that there may exist certain, pre-set, specifically linguistic strategies for the acquisition of language structures. A study of the acquisition of certain features of a particular linguistic structure by using new forms containing nonsense words has recently been reported (Cromer, 1975). The study was made on normal and educationally subnormal children, and also on normal adults. One particular strategy used by the normal children in dealing with the new instances of this structure appeared to coincide with the kind of behaviour which would be predicted if answers were given in accordance with some universally observed language patterns. Educationally subnormal children behaved not like the normal children, but like normal adults. The explanation for this finding was thought to be related to the fact that the subnormal children had been matched with the normal children on the basis of their mental age; they were, therefore, chronologically older and beyond a critical period for language learning when such strategies were likely to be employed. That is, neither the educationally subnormal children nor normal adults made use of the language-related strategy which was observed in many of the normal children. There is very little experimental work on other possible specifically linguistic strategies for language acquisition.

A slightly different approach might be to consider the 'content' of the language acquisition device. In this hypothesis, the child is believed to possess certain linguistic structures to which he attempts to match linguistic input. A related possibility is that certain linguistic structures are 'natural' and are easily acquired; they are structures which are found universally or near universally in the languages of the world. The brain, in other words, is thought to be 'pre-wired' to deal with certain types of specifically linguistic input. If there is any truth in these claims, the study of the linguistic structures of people suffering from damage to the language areas of the brain might provide clues to the nature of the intact language acquisition device. A few recent studies have begun to look at the language of adult dysphasic patients in terms of more modern linguistic theory, some with the intention of examining the way in which the grammar is actually represented in a speaker's brain. Myerson and Goodglass (1972) attempted to describe the language output of three patients with Broca dysphasia by the methods of transformational grammar. The three patients were differentially impaired. Myerson and Goodglass found an inverse correlation between the severity of the dysphasia and the number of specific types of distinctions that could be made in the base component, as well as in the number and types of rules which were used to generate surface structures. In some cases (e.g. negation, number of base-generated constituents which could actually be expressed in any utterance, etc.) the limitations seemed to parallel the order of acquisition by the child.

Schnitzer (1974) used methods of modern linguistic analysis in studying the language and grammatical judgements of a dysphasic patient. English sentences and non-sentences were read to the patient, and his task was to judge whether they were grammatical or not. His judgements generally agreed with those of normal individuals, but he did make several systematic errors. Overall, he judged certain exceptionally long, embedded, or conjoined grammatical sentences to be ungrammatical. In terms of specific structures, almost all of his incorrect judgements were related to three linguistic features: the absence of copula verbs, the absence of the subjects of sentences, and the absence of determiners. Some examples will make each category clear. The absence of the copula verb, 'to be', was noted in such sentences in his spontaneous speech as 'He mad', 'I scared', and 'They not fast'. In addition, sentences which were read to him with the copula omitted, such as 'The dog sick', and 'The pen coloured green', were judged by him to be grammatically correct. Similarly, he omitted subjects in his spontaneous speech ('Getting hungry', 'Got a good sleep last night') and judged sentences lacking subjects ('Kicked and punched', 'Walked about fifteen miles') to be grammatical. The same pattern occurred with determiners. Thus, he often omitted 'a' or 'the' ('Population is getting big', 'Almost lost game') in his own speech, and judged sentences without them ('Dog ate grass', 'Dog is in yard') to be grammatical. Schnitzer noted, however, that these forms were only omitted when the sentences did not carry new semantic information or where new information was marked by elements found elsewhere in the sentence. In sentences where the information was of a purely grammatical kind, Schnitzer's patient ignored the grammatical elements. For example, a series of relative clauses such as 'The man who went to the store' and 'The pig that lives in the pen' were judged by him to be fully grammatical sentences. Notice that they are also grammatical when the relative pronoun is omitted. The information which the relative pronoun conveys is syntactic – that this structure is a relative clause embedded on the noun which begins it. Schnitzer concludes that linguists have much to learn from such an analysis. In this case, for example, he claims that grammars ought to provide a way of representing the distinction between syntax and semantics. He feels that the grammars proposed by linguists should be conditioned by knowledge of the actual way in which grammar is represented in speakers' brains. Looked at the other way round, however, it may help to explain the linguistic disorders observed in dysphasic patients.

The problem is that the 'grammars' of adult dysphasic patients are many and varied. Instead of providing clues to the nature of the 'cause' of the language disorder, they merely reflect what occurs when a specified area of the brain is damaged. Language, by whatever means it is acquired, may be predominantly organised in particular areas of the brain. Lesions in these areas produce various kinds of dysphasia. By contrast, the study of developmental dysphasia, of children who possess normal cognitive capacities but who do not easily acquire language, may provide clues to the nature of the language acquisition device by providing evidence of the types of linguistic structures these children find difficult or impossible to master regardless of the mode of input.

Some 'Language-system' Experiments on Dysphasic Children

There has been a great deal of interest, in the past few years, in the supposed uniqueness of language in human beings. Obviously other animals have their own cognitive systems and display various types of intelligent behaviour. But many theorists have argued that only humans have the capacity for 'true language'. What is meant by 'true language' is not, however, entirely clear. Furthermore, the difficulty of studying 'language' in other species has often been compounded by the problem of choosing means of communication which the animal can handle. Since language functions should transcend particular modalities, it is possible to design systems which other animals may adequately use, but which still give evidence for the possession of these functions. There are really two issues involved here. One is whether non-human animals are capable of using linguistic functions, and the other is the extent to which linguistic functions can be shown in a non-auditory modality. The first issue is outside the scope of this chapter and it will be mentioned only peripherally. It only becomes important insofar as the techniques developed for studying communication in other species may be of use in helping to throw light on the abilities and deficiencies of children with developmental dysphasia. One important point must be emphasised: language functions and cognitive meanings are not identical. To state that an individual possesses a certain type of intelligence and is capable of understanding and making use of symbols for various contents and relations in the world, cannot tell us whether or how he is capable of expressing or understanding those meanings in a linguistic system. This point has been discussed elsewhere (see Cromer, 1974, 1976). Indeed, as we will later discover, dysphasic children and adults are capable of many types of complicated thought processes while being unable to understand or express them in a language system.

In 1969, Premack attempted to teach a type of language to Sarah, a chimpanzee. In order to do this, he avoided the aural/oral system and only employed materials that chimpanzees would be able to manipulate. Thus, he used a number of plastic symbols with a metal backing which would adhere to a magnetic board. Using operant conditioning techniques, he trained Sarah in the use of these materials. Each plastic nonsense shape was associated with a particular stimulus. Note that although Premack employed reinforcement techniques and gradually shaped the chimpanzee's behaviour, he did not claim that this was the way in which 'language' is normally acquired by humans. His interest was only to investigate whether or not language functions could be established in a chimpanzee in the absence of speech. Premack found that Sarah was able to acquire the basic communication units that he taught. These included the names for objects, various verbs describing actions, and modifiers, negation, and questions. Some of these consisted of judgements and communication of concepts as complicated as 'same' and 'different', and 'yes' and 'no'. For example, the chimpanzee was able to learn to place the symbol for 'same' between two like objects, and also between the name of the object and the object itself. Similarly, she was able to learn to place the symbol for 'not same' between unlike objects. Once this ability was acquired, she was able to indicate with the symbols for 'yes' and 'no' when these relations were used correctly. If the message placed on the board was (X) (same as) (X) or (X) (not same as) (Y), followed by the symbol for 'question', Sarah would reply with the symbol for 'yes'. And when messages like (X) (not same as) (X) or (X) (same as) (Y) were shown, she would reply with the symbol for 'no'. Premack was even able to teach Sarah hierarchical structures built up over time from simpler structures. Thus, starting from the simple sentence-instruction, 'Sarah insert banana pail, Sarah insert apple dish', Sarah was trained to carry out, without errors, the two instructions of inserting the banana into the pail and the apple into the dish, with the more condensed instructions, 'Sarah insert banana pail insert apple dish' and finally 'Sarah insert banana pail apple dish', in which the second uses of 'Sarah' and 'insert' were progressively eliminated.

Some writers have concluded that chimpanzees have been able to learn subject-verb-object strings, and indeed in Premack's experiment they appear to have done so. But again caution must be used in making such an interpretation. The terms 'subject', 'verb', and 'object' are linguistic, and are often used to express the meanings 'actor', 'action', and 'object', but they need not do so, and may not do so in the majority of sentences actually used by speakers. For example, although the subject of a sentence may be an actor or agent as in 'John hit the ball', subjects may serve a variety of other functions as well. In 'The key opened the door', the subject 'key' is an instrument, not an actor or agent. In 'John received a blow on the head', the subject 'John' is a patient. In 'John received a gift', 'John' is a recipient. In 'London is windy', the subject 'London' is a location. Indeed, this is the whole point of case grammar. Case grammatical conceptions express certain meanings more directly. Notions like 'subject' however, express a different level of generalisation, and one which is more purely grammatical. It has been argued by some researchers (e.g. Bowerman, 1973) that very young children's grammars are more adequately described in terms of a case grammar. Bowerman also notes, however, that at some point in development it appears necessary to invoke grammatical notions such as 'subject' and 'object' in order to account for the more purely linguistic transformations which are observed. It is not necessary to examine the merits of opposing theories of grammar merely in order to re-emphasise that, at least in some theories, grammatical meanings (such as 'subject') are not identical with specific cognitive meanings (such as 'actor'). It may be that the systems taught to chimpanzees are communication systems encoding the linkage of meanings rather than of linguistic elements. That is, it may be more accurate to describe some of the chimpanzee sentences in terms such as 'actor-action-acted upon' rather than 'subject-verb-object'. And this may be a crucial distinction when one considers dysphasia, in which cognitive meanings may be preserved whilst the more purely linguistic structures in which these are usually encoded break down. One possibility is that such artificial 'languages' can be learned by dysphasics precisely because they are not 'linguistic'.

Glass *et al.* (1973) demonstrated that a communication system based on Premack's system for the chimpanzee could be learned by patients with global dysphasia resulting from cerebral vascular accidents. Seven patients were trained in the use of a system employing cut-out paper symbols for words. The paper symbols varied in colour, size, and shape, were functionally equivalent to words, and were arranged in a left-right direction on a table. Glass *et al.* (1973) reported that all seven patients, taking on average one month of training, successfully learned same/different and interrogative constructions. In addition, two of the patients were able to learn simple sentences consisting of what were described as 'subject-verb-direct-object' strings. They were able to produce and comprehend such sentences at an approximate level of accuracy of 80 per cent. There was evidence that the other five patients would also have progressed to that level had training been continued, but for administrative reasons this was not possible (e.g. some patients were discharged from the hospital, etc.). Glass *et al.* (1973) concluded that global aphasics may not suffer a cognitive impairment which is in direct proportion to their linguistic impairment, and that rather sophisticated and abstract symbolic thought can be carried out by patients with severe language deficits. What is the case of children with developmental or early acquired dysphasia? Might it be that they have the cognitive ability to learn such a communication system despite their deficient or almost non-existent language? The teachers and staff at schools for dysphasic children have no doubts that their children are capable of extremely sophisticated symbolic thought. As we shall show, the teachers are correct in their assessment.

Hughes (1972, 1974/1975) carried out a study (following a suggestion of Dr B. M. Hermelin) designed to discover whether children diagnosed as dysphasic could acquire the type of communication system that Premack had used with chimpanzees. The four children she studied were cases of developmental or early acquired dysphasia. These subjects were part of a special group of children with normal or above normal intelligence as measured on non-verbal tests, but who were unable to comprehend or produce language. Hughes trained the four children individually in half-hour sessions, twice weekly for about nine weeks, using materials similar to those Premack had employed – i.e. plastic shapes with a metal backing which were placed on a magnetic board. She reported that the dysphasic children rapidly acquired all of the functions taught. These included the names of various objects and persons, verbs such as 'give' and 'point to', direct and indirect objects, negatives, modifiers, and questions. Thus, like the global aphasics mentioned earlier, these children were able to acquire a fairly sophisticated communication system without difficulty. The crucial question now becomes: why are children without language able to acquire Premack's system? There are a number of possibilities. One is that this system, although a communication system, is not a 'language' in the sense in which linguists would define language. This argument, however, contains a logical fallacy which becomes particularly obvious when applied as a criticism to the research on communication systems in chimpanzees. The argument usually begins with the assertion that only human beings have language. When chimpanzees are shown to be able to acquire one or another analogue of language, it is then argued that the system under consideration is not really 'language' since, by definition, chimpanzees are not capable of language. On the other hand, in the experiments just reviewed, various human groups were trained on just such a communication system. In one group, the known language ability of a group of adults had been impaired as a consequence of a stroke. That they could acquire 'Premackese' in spite of their linguistic impairment is certainly significant. Similarly, the dysphasic children either never developed language or lost what language abilities they had at an early age. They too were able to acquire the Premack system easily. This in fact could also suggest that the argument put forward by the linguists is after all correct; it may be that Premackese, while encoding some of the functions that language encodes, is, nevertheless, not really the same as a linguistic system, even when it adequately serves as a communication system. That is, it bears little resemblance to natural language; it utilises only simple ordering rules, and has no transformations; and it does not really constitute a generative system.

There is another possibility, however, which needs consideration. It may be that the impairment in dysphasics is purely auditory in nature. This argument would hold that the Premack system presents little difficulty to dysphasic individuals because it is a visual system. In order to test this possibility, we designed a study (Barna, 1975) in which children with early acquired dysphasia were given instruction in a system analogous to that of Premack, but which was presented in the auditory modality. In order to carry out this study, an apparatus was built which consisted of 15 cassette playback tape recorders operated by two keyboards, one controlled by the researcher and the other controlled by the dysphasic child. Each keyboard had 15 buttons arranged in three rows of five. Pressing a key operated a particular recorder. Each recorder had a special looped tape with a repeating sound or noise, so that pressing one of the buttons immediately produced that particular sound. With the two keyboards, either the child or the researcher could produce a series of sounds by successively pressing a series of buttons. The original intention was to examine both production and comprehension. After training in the acquisition of particular sounds to stand for particular objects and actions (establishment of 'words'), sequences such as 'Sara point-to car' and 'Monkey insert car dish' could be produced. For example, the experimenter might point to the car, and the child would be expected to encode this action into the appropriate sequences of noises which stood for this, 'Sara point-to car'. In a comprehension task, the researcher would produce the series of noises, and the child would carry out the actions, thereby indicating his understanding of the series. For example, the child hearing the sequence of signals 'Monkey insert car dish' would have to show the monkey inserting the car into the dish. In practice, however, it was virtually impossible to elicit any productive responses by the dysphasic children since they were unwilling to manipulate the control panel. Indeed, they could not be induced to construct a sequence of even two sounds. Consequently, the experimental training developed primarily into the comprehension task, rather than using both comprehension and production as Premack, and later Hughes, had done.

Four children, all with acquired dysphasia, took part in the training programme. These children had IQs within the normal range, only minimal hearing loss, but had either no verbal language or language at a rudimentary level. Their ages at the time of onset of the disability, which occurred in all of them without known traumatic injury, were $2\frac{1}{2}$, $4\frac{1}{2}$, $4\frac{1}{2}$, and 7 years. At the time of the study, three of the children were between 9 and 10 years old, and the fourth was 13.

Experiments by Eimas (see Eimas, 1974) have shown that perception of speech differs from the perception of nonspeech acoustic signals as early as one month of age. Since these appear to be processed in different ways, it was decided that two types of signal should be used on the tapes. Thus, two of the children heard only noises for their signals, while the other two heard only speech-like sounds. The noises were produced by various instruments including bells, rattles, squeakers, and two musical instruments – a recorder and a xylophone. The speech-like sounds were chosen in consultation with the children's speech therapist and were based on a set of phonemes which the child could actually say.

Due to scheduling difficulties, we were unable to extend the learning situations to nine weeks in order to parallel the length of time used by Hughes with the visual material. Therefore, many of the more advanced structures were not attempted since these relied on the knowledge of simpler structures which were just being acquired by the end of the five-week period of the present study. The children in Hughes' study were given between 11 and 15 half-hour training sessions; in the present study they had 8 to 10 half-hour sessions. Despite the fact that only simpler structures were eventually attempted with most of the children, the results offer some interesting clues as to the possible nature of the disorder. The first function that it is necessary to establish is that of the 'word'. This was initially done by giving the child a toy to play with, and then taking it back and holding it up while producing the corresponding sound which was to be its name. After a short time the researcher would produce the sound and the child had to hold up the appropriate toy, out of a set of toys. In a similar fashion the children were trained with 'words' for actions such as 'give' and 'point-to'. In each session, there were specific blocks of testing. The criterion for rating a language function as having been acquired was for the child to have demonstrated at least 70 per cent correct usage in the block of testing. All four children learned the symbols for at least six nouns and four verbs. In addition, three of the four subjects learned the symbols for their own name and that of the researcher. It is clear, then, that for all four children it was possible to establish the 'word' function. These particular dysphasic children were clearly capable of forming links between sound and meaning despite the fact that two of the children had been labelled as having 'auditory agnosia'. The findings of this study do not support a theory of a generalised or global word deafness. On the other hand, Barna (1975) reported that all four children showed some perceptual difficulty. The children appeared to have more trouble in discriminating the sounds than one would expect from normal listeners; they also appeared to need to concentrate their attention all the time. One child had an apparent inability to discriminate between different sounds of the same type. For example, he was unable to discriminate between the sounds of two toy horns even though they varied greatly in pitch. Similarly, he could not discriminate between a high and low recorder note. The children appeared to try to make use of visual cues whenever possible, so that performance was better when actual noise makers were used or else when the sounds were uttered (offering the possibility of lip reading) than when the same noises or sounds were presented on the tape equipment. In addition, three of the subjects displayed great variability in their responses both during and between sessions. This was seen not only for the 'word' function, but for other functions as well. Nevertheless, in spite of these difficulties, all four children were able to establish a vocabulary of at least ten 'words'.

Attempts were made to teach the children simple sentences of the so-called 'subject-verb-object' type. The aim was to build up the sentences word by word, beginning with two element strings such as 'Give doll' and 'Point-to cat'. Eventually three element strings such as 'Monkey point-to cat', would be attempted. In fact, the two element stage constituted the ceiling of learning for three of the four children. Only the child who mastered three element strings was given any training on longer structures and on more complex functions. This child acquired not only three element strings, but went on to acquire four element (subject)-(verb)-(direct object)-(indirect object) strings. In a final session in which normal speech rather than the experimental procedure was used, this same child also acquired the functions of class concepts, and questions. Negation was also taught to this child and while she displayed some acquisition, her performance on this function did not reach the required criterion.

What can we conclude from these preliminary results? Our main purpose was to see whether the Premack-type language functions which Hughes had been able to establish with dysphasic children could also be acquired by four other dysphasic children at the same school, when the material was presented in the auditory rather than the visual modality. There were large discrepancies between the results of the present study and that carried out by Hughes. On the other hand, in the Hughes study, the average number of sessions per child was twelve, whereas in this study it was only nine. Thus, one can only speculate as to the possible outcome had the degree of training been equal. One child was clearly close to acquiring the complete set of functions that Hughes had previously taught. Barna reports that a second child was also showing distinct progress when training was terminated. But the other two subjects showed little improvement from session to session, and Barna claimed that it was quite unlikely that their performance would have reached beyond the results obtained. Examination of these limited accomplishments, however, may nevertheless provide some clues.

It is important to note that the four children who were studied did not constitute a homogeneous group. They differed greatly in their ability to acquire the structures on which training was attempted; but there was no indication that any differences between the subjects was attributable to their training with noises or speech-like sounds. Despite this problem, however, some conclusions can be drawn. Firstly, all of the children were able to link sound with meaning; all four children acquired a vocabulary of at least ten 'words'. Secondly, three of the four children were able to acquire two element strings. This might be taken as evidence that neither their memory for auditory information nor their ability to sequence sounds was as impaired as some theories would appear to suggest. But the fact that they performed worse on this task than the children in Hughes study using visual symbols leaves the question unanswered.

There is yet another way to approach the problem. Children with devolopmental and acquired dysphasia are given instruction in reading and writing in their schools. Although these children are essentially without language in that they do not produce or comprehend *spoken* language, they do acquire writing skills and are able, after a great deal of instruction, to write letters to their parents, and to produce written descriptions and stories. As might be expected, these productions usually contain many grammatical errors. On the other hand, the early written productions by deaf children, who are also learning language 'through the eye' also contain many grammatical errors. An analysis of written material gathered in controlled conditions from dysphasic and from deaf children may reveal whether these two groups differ in the kinds of errors they make. If the underlying deficit in dysphasic children is specifically auditory in nature, then their errors should be similar to those made by the deaf. If these errors differ, however, their analysis may provide clues as to the nature of the dysphasic deficit.

A Study of the Writings of Dysphasic and Deaf Children

In order to study errors in written materials, it is necessary to know what the writer is attempting to communicate. Without this knowledge, sentences which appear to be well formed may in fact be quite disordered. If we merely read the sentence, 'The boy talked to the girl and went upstairs', it appears perfectly grammatical. But if we know that it was the girl who went upstairs, then we are dealing with a sentence in which the writer does not know how to construct the complex sentence involving a change of subject and substitution of pronoun to convey the precise information, i.e. 'The boy talked to the girl and she went upstairs'. In the writings of dysphasic children it is not always possible to know what the child is attempting to communicate. In a preliminary analysis of letters written to their parents, it was virtually impossible to analyse the structure of the sentences since the intended meaning was often unknown and unclear. It was therefore necessary to set up controlled situations for the children to describe. In addition, with situations experimentally controlled, it is possible to design specific stories which could encourage various types of sentence production.

To this end, stories were designed and presented as puppet shows or were acted out with small toy animals. Here, only the story for which the writings have been analysed will be described. Four hand puppets were employed – a wolf, a monkey, and two ducks. Having two animals of the same type introduces the possibility of plurals; also, by designing the story so that those two characters would be in conflict, the child must somehow differentiate between them, and this would necessitate the use of adjectives, relative clauses, and other linguistic entities. In addition, the materials were chosen with a view to eliciting the largest possible differentiation. Two wire containers were used, one tall and narrow, the other low and wide. The size of the containers was such that they could hold table-tennis (ping-pong) balls, and they were modelled to look like oversize versions of the beakers used in typical Piagetian conservation experiments. The action of the puppet show must be described in order to understand the writings produced by the children.

At the beginning of the presentation, the low, wide container held eight balls, while the tall, narrow container was empty. The wolf, alone in view, looks at the two containers and then grasps one of the balls in his mouth and transfers it to the tall container. He transfers a second ball in this way and then stands back and looks at the two containers again. Next, he successively places two more balls in the tall container. At this point the monkey comes into view, bites the wolf on the ear and generally creates a nuisance; finally the wolf chases the monkey away. A duck then appears on the scene and decides to undo what the wolf has done by tipping all the balls back from the tall container into the low one. The duck then leaves. The wolf returns, and with movements meant to imply exasperation, goes through the same sequence as before: moving one ball at a time into the tall container, pausing in between to view the beakers. Again, just as he finishes transferring the fourth ball, the monkey re-appears and again annoys the wolf and bites him on the ear, and once again the wolf chases the monkey off-stage. (The repetition was designed to bring out adverbial phrases such as 'again', 'a second time', and to force the child to explain a repeating sequence of actions.) The duck again returns and again tips the balls from the tall into the low container, but this time is interrupted by a second duck, of somewhat different appearance. This second duck takes the side of the wolf and tries to prevent the first duck from pouring the balls back into the wide container. They fight. The wolf returns, and mistaking the two ducks as being against him, chases them away. (The story was designed to elicit some degree of differentiation, not only in terms of physical appearance, for instance of the two containers and the two ducks, but also in terms of motivations.)

Children were tested in their classrooms in groups of six to ten. Their own classroom teacher carefully explained to them that they were going to see a puppet show and that they should first just watch it. Then, they would write down what they saw. The teacher was able to communicate with the dysphasic children through a mixture of repetition and gesture. The puppets were introduced as, 'Here is a wolf. Here is a monkey. Here is a duck. Here is another duck.' This was the only verbal interaction during the whole of the show. At the same time, the teacher listed, on the blackboard: a wolf, a monkey, a duck, a duck. Thus in addition to the four names, the children were provided with the indefinite article 'a', and orally, they heard the frame 'Here is . . .' and once, the quantifier adjective 'another'. The children were allowed to write for as long as they liked; this was generally for about half an hour to 45 minutes. During this period, children would sometimes ask their teacher for help, usually with the spelling of words, which was communicated to the dysphasic group by means of finger spelling against the palm of the hand. The teacher provided only the spelling of the word asked for and in the grammatical form requested by the child.

The main aim was to compare the writings of dysphasic children with those of deaf children. In this preliminary analysis, the results from a group of receptive-expressive dysphasic children will be compared with the writings obtained, using the same story, from profoundly, congenitally deaf children. The medical records indicated that four of the group of the ten dysphasic children had never possessed language, and they will be referred to here as the developmental aphasic group. The remaining six children had developed some language function, but this deteriorated in later years. The ages of onset of language deterioration in these six children were 2 years 6 months, 2 years 9 months, 4 years, 4 years 6 months, 5 years, and 7 years. The ages of the ten children at the time of testing ranged from 7 years 6 months to 16 years, with a median age of 13 years 6 months. Their non-verbal IQs on the Collins-Drever test were in the normal range, with the exception of one child whose IQ was 75, and another with an IQ of 135. The range of the remaining IQs was 93 to 116, and the overall median IQ of the group was 99.5.

Of the ten children, two merely drew pictures or copied the names of the animals from the blackboard. These were the two youngest children (7 years 6 months and 10 years), and one was in the developmental group whilst the other was in the group of acquired dysphasia. Two other children produced written samples which were so severely disordered that a grammatical analysis cannot be attempted. Again, one of the writings was by a child with developmental dysphasia, and the other by a child with acquired dysphasia. The story one of the children wrote will serve as an example of the difficulty in interpretation or analysis. Several children used the word 'basket' to refer to the low container and the word 'tube' to refer to the tall, narrow one. Punctuation and capitalisation are the child's:

> table tennis ball tube putting
>   basket bite in a wolf down.
> the buck [*Note:* probably reversed letter, intending 'duck'] tube
>   look and fritened the to you cause over basket.
> In monkey sad CDMD here you no?
> In duck no over duck two tennis ball down on happy
> In to wolf see look duck duck angry wolf bad
> quck good duck happy two on over no wolf you

Elimination of the two severely disorganised samples left a total of six to analyse – two from children with developmental dysphasia and four from children with acquired dysphasia at ages 2 years 6 months, 2 years 9 months, 4 years, and 7 years.

For a preliminary analysis, the productions of a class of six congenitally profoundly deaf children were chosen for comparison. The range of ages of these six children was 9 years 11 months to 10 years 8 months with a median age of between 10 years 5 months and 10 years 6 months. The range of IQs was 80 to 123, with a median IQ of 101·5. Hearing loss varied from 90 to 120 dBs. All six children produced material that could be analysed. A few children in other classrooms produced drawings or a list of the animal names as two of the dysphasic children had done, but these were all younger children. None of the deaf children produced the severely disorganised language similar to that quoted above.

At first glance, the productions of the six dysphasic children and the six deaf children do not appear to differ in any distinct way. Indeed, by only reading a story produced by either a deaf or a dysphasic child, it would be difficult to identify the group to which the child belonged. Below there are two stories, and the reader may wish to identify which is written by a deaf and which by a dysphasic child.

I

The wolf picked up ball to put the basket. The monkey bite the woof ear. The woof said, 'Woof! wog!' The wolf chased the monkey. Suddenly coming the duck to pick up the basket and dropped the ball. Suddenly the wolf coming but the wolf surprised. The wolf was very angy because the ball is gone. The wolf picked up the ball again. Suddenly the monkey coming and to bite the wolf's ear again. The wolf chased the monkey again. Coming the two ducks to picked up the basket dropped the ball to a small basket but the two ducks are frighted. The wolf was very angry the monkey but the poor monkey the wolf bite the monkey. The monkey died.

II

The wolf is taking his table tennis ball. he is putting in the tube. The monkey is bitting the wolf's ear.
       chasing
The wolf is running* the monkey. The duck is taking round the tube. The ball is in the basket. The wolf is saying oh gone the ball. again the wolf is taking his table tennis ball in the tube. The monkey is bitting the wolf's ear. The wolf is chasing him.
    The duck is saying oh again ball in the tube. The duck is bitting the duck's ear.

* The word 'chasing' was written above the word 'running', as if the child had second thoughts and changed the latter for the former.

There are clearly a great number of grammatical errors in both of these productions; and not many readers would be able to identify with confidence that (I) was written by a deaf child and (II) by a dysphasic. Closer analysis, however, reveals some important differences.

It is not possible to make a transformational analysis on the basis of so small a sample of sentences. It is impossible to see which structures might be interrelated unless one is able to survey a very large number of sentences. In addition, there is the problem that children may be capable of producing other grammatical structures, although these were not present in this story.

The views relative to the omissions of certain grammatical structures can therefore only be tentative until further research is carried out. On the other hand, grammatical errors – errors of commission – may reveal those aspects of language with which the child encounters specific difficulty. That is to say, at this point it is not possible to delineate what are the difficulties of the dysphasic child in encoding particular meanings in the linguistic code. One can note, however, the types of sentences, the types of meanings and of structural types which were attempted, and also those types which were not attempted by the children. The writings were analysed in several different ways, and the results cited here are a summary of the significant differences observed between the deaf and dysphasic productions.

It was not difficult in most cases to divide the structures into sentence units. Usually the child himself has provided the punctuation which indicates his divisions. In only one case were a large number of arbitrary decisions required. This was a deaf child who connected his entire production with a series of 'ands'. The deaf, in general, wrote slightly longer stories than the dysphasics, but when a count was made of the mean number of words per sentence, deaf and the dyphasics performed similarly, the deaf with an average of 7·76 words per sentence and the dysphasics with 7.61. The language of the dysphasic children, however, under close analysis, is in fact quite different. In terms of word counts this difference is reflected not in the number of words per sentence, which was the same in the two groups, but in the number of categories per sentence. By categories is meant entities such as noun phrases, verb phrases, adverbial phrases, etc. In these terms, the dysphasic language shows itself to be less complex than that produced by the deaf. The deaf, on average, produced 4·51 categories per sentence, whilst the dysphasics produced only 3·73, a difference which was statistically significant (p < ·01).

What linguistic structures are affected by this lack of complexity? One obvious difference between the groups was that a few dysphasic children seemed to repeat a single sentence type with which they were familiar. One child, for example, simply produced a list of ten sentences, nine of which used the present progressive: 'The wolf is getting the balls. The duck is looking at the balls. The wolf is catching the monkey. The monkey is catching the wolf.', etc. The deaf, by contrast, appeared to try a number of different sentence types and these included different categories of verb tense. One possible count is therefore the number of different verb types used by each child. Verbs were categorised into seven traditional categories: present, past, future, copulas, progressives, perfects, and infinitives. A child was credited with attempting a category even if he made errors in doing so. The children in the dysphasic group never attempted verbs in the present, future, (i.e. verb with the auxiliary 'will' or ''ll'), or any of the perfect tenses; but each of the above categories was attempted by at least one deaf child. The fact that no dysphasic child attempted those verb types in his story could be accounted for, however, by the small size of the sample. It is nevertheless possible to compare the variety of verb types used by each child. Deaf children attempted an average of 3·33 different verb types in their sentences. Dysphasic children only had an average of 2·16 different verb types. This difference was again statistically significant ($p < ·02$).

Not only did the use of verb tenses differ, but there was a difference in the use of certain traditional linguistic structure types. Numbers are too small to carry out the usual tests of significance, but it was noted that no dysphasic child produced sentences with negatives; no questions were used; and there were virtually no complement clause structures (although one child attempted one such sentence). In addition, the dysphasic children never used a qualifying adjective. By contrast, three of the six deaf children used negatives, two used questions, and four used complement clauses. Four deaf children also used a total of 11 qualifying adjectives. It must be emphasised again that these differences are only tentative. In the story which was quoted earlier, and which could not be analysed, the question mark symbol was used by this particular dysphasic child, although it is impossible to tell with certainty whether any kind of question was intended. Also, it would be surprising if negatives were not present in other writings of the dysphasic children, even if they have trouble forming negative sentences without errors.

In spite of these apparent differences in some of the categories used, the real interest lies not here, but in the analysis of errors. In fact, error analysis on most sentence types revealed that the deaf usually made a greater number of errors – (this was because they attempted more sentence types). The dysphasic writings, on the other hand, had fewer errors, but this was due to the fact that the children did not attempt a variety of structures. The question one can reasonably ask in this respect is: What determines the nature of the omissions? We have already seen that the sentences produced by dysphasic children, although of identical length to those of the deaf, contain fewer grammatical categories.

Furthermore, dysphasic children generally wrote only simple sentences – often the various kinds of simple sentences they had been taught. Deaf children seemed far more able to combine sentence types which include additional transformations. A count was carried out of the total number of sentences which included one or more embedded or conjoined structures as opposed to sentences without these. A few examples will make these counts clearer. Sentences rated as having one conjoined structure would include: 'Suddenly the wolf coming but the wolf surprised' and 'The wolf was very angry because the ball is gone'. An example with two embedded or conjoined elements would be 'Suddenly coming the duck to picked up the basket and dropped the ball'. Only 12·0 per cent of the sentences produced by dysphasic children had one or more embedded or conjoined structure, as compared to 35·9 per cent of the sentences produced by the deaf children. This difference was highly significant (p < ·001). It was also noticed that the rare sentences with an embedded or conjoined structure produced by dysphasic children often omitted the second verb, as in 'The monkey is frightened because a wolf bad'. No dysphasic child attempted sentences with more than one embedding or conjoining. The deaf, in contrast, produced sentences of which 10·9 per cent had two or more embedded or conjoined elements. This difference between the two groups was again significant (p < ·01).

The simplicity of the dysphasic children's writings was not restricted to the omission of complex sentences. It was also reflected in the lack of transformational structure within simple sentences; thus they never linked two adjectives (e.g. 'the big, tall one'; 'He is big and strong') whereas adjective linking occurred in some of the deaf children's stories. The dysphasics never produced adverb-adjective strings (such as 'the very big ball'); again, these occurred in some of the samples of the deaf children. Conjunctions were rarely used by the dysphasic children even internally, as for instance in the linking of two noun phrases within a simple sentence, and they virtually never used them to combine two independent clauses. The deaf by contrast produced many conjunctions, some of these linking two independent clauses.

It is of interest to turn back to the two samples printed earlier. My guess is that, at first glance, most readers will have found difficulty in deciding which story was written by the deaf child and which by the dysphasic child. But now, in the light of the statistical analyses which have just been given, it should be fairly easy to see how those two written productions differ. The first, that written by a profoundly deaf child, contains a variety of verb tenses, although he doesn't attempt to use the simple present tense.*

---

* 'Bite' was not considered as a present tense since analysis revealed that many children who clearly use past tenses in other situations, spelled 'bit' (past tense) with a final 'e'.

The deaf child uses copula verbs in both present and past ('are frighted', 'is gone', 'was very angry'), simple past tense forms ('chased', 'dropped', 'picked up', 'died', 'said'), progressive forms ('coming'), and infinitives ('to bite', 'to pick up'). The dysphasic child (story II) uses only progressives with the present tense auxiliary ('is taking', 'is putting', 'is bitting', 'is running', 'is saying', 'is chasing') and one copula verb in the present tense ('is'). The deaf child uses several types of coordinate structures, including those in which the subject remained the same ('the wolf coming but the wolf surprised', 'coming the two ducks to picked up the basket dropped the ball but the two duck are frighted'), and those in which the subjects differed ('the wolf was very angry because the ball is gone'). The dysphasic child uses no coordinate constructions. Furthermore he wrote two sentences in which there was one embedded or conjoined structure, but omitted the second verb in both cases ('The wolf is saying oh gone the ball', 'The duck is saying oh again ball in the tube'); also there are no examples of sentences with two or more embedded or conjoined structures. By contrast, the deaf child's story contains six sentences which had one embedded or conjoined structure, and two which had two or more ('Suddenly coming the duck to pick up the basket and dropped the ball', 'Coming the two ducks to picked up the basket dropped the ball to a small basket but the two duck are frighted'). The deaf child also uses complement verbs ('picked up ball to put . . .', 'coming the duck to pick up . . .', etc.), which are lacking in the dysphasic child's production. Overall, the deaf child has an average of 5·15 categories per sentence, compared to 3·5 for the dysphasic. In these particular samples, the deaf child also has longer sentences (an average of 8·6 words per sentence compared to the dysphasic child's 7·4), although for the group as a whole the mean sentence lengths did not differ. Additional complexity in sentence structure is shown by the deaf child in that he uses nine adjectives including two qualifying adjectives ('small', 'poor') (totally lacking in any of the dysphasic writings) and predicate adjectives (e.g. 'is gone', 'are frighted', 'surprised', 'angry'). There were also seven uses of adverbs ('suddenly', 'again', 'very'), and even an adverb-adjective string ('very angry'). The dysphasic child used three adverbs ('gone', 'again'), but no adjectives, and consequently no adjective-adjective or adverb-adjective combinations. The two written productions, which appeared on the surface to be similar, are, in fact, quite different in terms of the dimensions described. But what is different about the dysphasic writing? Is it merely less complex, or is it a special kind of complexity that is lacking? If so, could this latter give a clue to the nature of the underlying disability?

The Hypothesis of a Hierarchical Structuring Deficit

In an overall assessment of the written language abilities of the group of
dysphasic children that were studied, varying degrees of disorder were
noted. Thus, when the story was presented visually, there was a grammatical disorganisation in the output of these children. This disorganisation was at the level not of orthography but of the elements and categories
of the sentence. This observation, however, also applies to the writing of
congenitally deaf children who, like the dysphasic children, are learning
language 'by eye'. On the other hand, this preliminary analysis of writings
of the deaf and dysphasic children shows that their difficulties are indeed
quite different. The deaf children made more errors, but these were errors
of commission. They tried a variety of structures including many which
relied on complex transformations; in contrast, the dysphasic children
wrote simpler sentences and failed to use the kinds of structure that
would involve a true hierarchical organisation of the overall sentence.

One reason for the difference could be accounted for by the fact that the
children were from different schools, and have not been exposed to the
same teaching methods. (For instance, the dysphasic children had experience with Lea's colour pattern scheme (1970) which is especially
designed to help children with language disorders.) There are reasons,
however, which suggest that the differences between the dysphasic and
deaf groups were not related to particular differences in teaching materials.
Firstly, dysphasic children are exposed to a type of language which is as
complex in structure as the one used with deaf children; secondly, and
more important, language samples collected from a group of children,
labelled as 'phonologically disabled' appear to be quite different from
those of the receptive-expressive dysphasic children, even though they
were from the same school and were exposed to the same teaching
methods.

It might have been expected that the dysphasic children's writings
would show difficulties with particular grammatical devices – e.g. the
formation of plurals, possessives, etc. In fact, this was not the case. It had
already been shown, in Hughes' extension of Premack's work, that dysphasic children possessed the cognitive functions encoded in language,
and were able to use these with the token symbol system. It is not surprising, then, that they should attempt to encode these same functions in
written language. What is interesting is that they did not make a significantly greater number of errors than the deaf on those grammatical
entities which they attempted.

Another possible expectation was that the dysphasic children's writings would display difficulties with word order, especially in view of the emphasis given to possible sequencing difficulties from which these children are said to suffer. These results, however, do not entirely invalidate the sequencing hypothesis. It should be recalled that two productions were so disorganised that analysis of grammatical constituents could not be attempted. But even if this be the case, the kind of difficulty in the sequential ordering of words is in fact quite different from that predicted by the experimental results usually cited in support of sequential deficit hypotheses. The difficulty displayed by the dysphasic children, even in the two disordered samples, is not at the phoneme or orthographical level, and it is also possible that their difficulties may result from a 'hierarchical' disability.

The productions of the remaining six dysphasic children lend support to the view that their problem with language lies in its hierarchical organisation. The dysphasic children's problem does not appear to be solely attributable to the increased difficulty found in the transformations involved in complex sentences. They also lacked the kinds of devices that allow any interruptions – e.g. the transformations required for the production of relative clauses, conjunctions joining two nouns or joining two verbs with the same subject, etc. But this conjecture, like those that have been criticised earlier, is also based on a current assumption, namely, that language is hierarchically organised. This assumption stems, in part, from Lashley's early paper (1951) in which he points out the problems and limitations that exist in conceiving several specific types of behaviour as sequentially ordered. His views have been echoed in the modern linguistic approach, proposed by Chomksy (1959, 1965, 1976), and basically supported by even those linguists who criticize other aspects of Chomksy's theory. One fundamental problem is to determine what is meant by 'hierarchical ordering'. This terminology is now in common use although it seems to have different connotations.

The most common use of the term refers to descriptions of behaviour, organised simultaneously at several levels of complexity. I am not referring here, however, to this use of the term 'hierarchical'. In the present context, 'hierarchical' refers to a type of process which must be assumed to exist if sequential behaviour is to be explained as organised, purposeful and meaningful. Pure sequential ordering or mere associative links between adjacent elements (including higher order associations) have been shown to be inadequate in explaining grammatical structures. The kind of hierarchical complexity that is meant here involves, for example, the analysis of a complex behaviour into its component parts in which the performance of some parts is postponed while performance of other parts takes priority; in the words of Miller and Chomsky (1963), 'One natural criterion might be the ability to interrupt one part of the performance until some other part has been completed.' Neisser (1967) has written about hierarchical complexity in terms of organised entities in which the individual parts derive their meaning from the whole structure. Sentence elements are interdependent and not all their interrelationships are equally strong. Such a view, applied to language behaviour, calls for the use of transformational devices which allow the reordering and interruption of surface structure features. This type of analysis is now often applied to the simple sentences which are produced by young children. But the written sentences which were produced by the dysphasic children included simple structures they had learnt. Thus, one major obstacle for the proponent of the hypothesis that dysphasic children suffer from a hierarchical ordering deficit is the presence in their writing of these simple sentences. It may be, however, that dysphasic children are actually using simple grammatical rules based on adjacent elements. That is, simple sentences written by normal children may, in fact, be evidence of hierarchically organised structures, but in dysphasic children they may merely be sequentially ordered. How might one determine this? One possibility would be to study dysphasic children in an attempt to find evidence of an inability to deal with certain transformations of an understood structure. Another possibility would be to determine whether, in their productions, they are unable to make sentence changes which require 'planning' of the utterance, so that tense or person agreement fails when the sequence is interrupted by other intervening material. A third approach would be to note whether grammatical structures which require hierarchical ordering are lacking in these children. One such structure would be the relative clause which requires interruption of one sequence by another, for example, 'The boy who was hurt was crying'. In their written productions, dysphasic children did not produce relative clauses. Even categories which seem to be merely sequential, such as the ordering of adjective sequences, may in fact be ordered in terms of a hierarchical principle. For example, it is more natural to speak of 'the two large black cats' than of 'the two black large cats', or of 'the black large two cats'. It was interesting to note that the children in the dysphasic group avoided using any qualifying adjectives. But, as has been emphasised, this study was merely a preliminary investigation of written sentence production and it is possible that the dysphasic children had the ability to produce some of these structures but merely failed to do so in the particular samples collected. The fact that their written language productions omitted the kinds of structure which are dependent on hierarchical organisation, whereas these occurred in the language samples from the deaf children, is thus merely suggestive. The hypothesis of a hierarchical ordering disability, however, is supported by a very different kind of evidence.

It may be recalled that, when reviewing the studies of the disabilities of dysphasic children, there was general agreement that these children lacked all sense of rhythm. They are unable to march in step, to clap to tunes, or to reproduce rhythmic sequences by tapping. Whereas many people might assume that rhythmic behaviour requires solely a serial chain of successive elements, Lashley (1951) has pointed out that a rhythmic pattern is in fact a single structural unit. Neisser (1967) elaborated this idea and claimed that rhythms provide sets of reference points to which digits and words can be attached. He claims that the limit of memory span may be determined by the capacity to organise extended rhythmic sequences. Neisser claims that if rhythm is viewed as a basic ability, it would help to explain such phenomena as the ability of subjects to know, when recalling a string of digits, the position of a specific digit in the series. It would also help to explain the difficulty of backward recall. According to Neisser, backward reproductions are difficult because they demand rearrangement of a rhythmic pattern. For example, I have often noticed that most people have trouble in working out mentally the name 'Franklin' if it is spelt backwards – N i l k n a r f. Nilknarf, when pronounced, induces a four-four letter pattern, and even when the letters are rearranged and are put in place it seems difficult to change to the five-three pattern required by Franklin. Neisser speculates that the processes of spoken language are continuous with those of active, verbal memory, both of them involving the synthesis of rhythmic patterns.

Martin (1972) presents the strongest case for the conceptualisation of rhythms as hierarchically structured units. It is a misconception, he claims, to believe that rhythms imply only periodic, repetitive behaviour. Rhythmic sequences possess, in fact, hierarchical organisation. The alternative – a series of elements that are successive or concatenated in time – cannot have a structured internal organisation. Martin suggests that such a view has important implications for the production of rhythmic sequences and spoken language. Indeed they would have important implications in the analysis of perceptual processes. For example, this hierarchical ability would allow input sounds to be temporally patterned. Furthermore, rhythmically patterned sounds have a time trajectory that allows them to be tracked without the necessity for continuous monitoring. That is, the perception of initial or early elements in the pattern would allow later occurring elements to be anticipated. This would give rise to efficient perceptual strategies. Martin claims that the alternative, the perception of merely concatenated sounds, would require continuous attention; and Kracke (1975) noted in her rhythm experiments that the dysphasic children attempted to do precisely that. In her experiment, mentioned previously, the children compared rhythmic sequences and were required to give same/different judgments. She reported that the normal and the deaf children used what she termed 'a Gestalt strategy': they appeared to try to perceive the patterns in a direct, unreflective way without concentrating on the individual elements. By contrast, the dysphasic children used what Kracke called an 'element-by-element' strategy; that is to say, they attempted to repeat the elements to themselves, one by one, before giving a judgment. She reports also that some children even tried to capture the rhythm by verbal labelling, as in 'lonn-lonn-shor' (i.e. long-long-short). In direct contrast to the usual view that dysphasic children have a sequencing disability, it may be possible to claim that they can cope with sequencing tasks, but it is important to bear in mind that unless the elements can be arranged in a rhythmic pattern nobody can in fact reproduce a sequence. Perkins (1974) has shown that normal adults use rhythmic hierarchies to code sequential positions, and Dooling (1974) demonstrated the importance of rhythm in the perception of speech. There are also observations derived from neurological studies suggesting the important role of rhythm in the language process. Robinson and Solomon (1974) claim that rhythmic patterns, unlike other non-speech auditory entities, are processed better by the same hemisphere which is dominant for speech. Dennis and Whitaker (1976), basing their conclusion on a study of left and right hemidecorticate children, reported that different configurations of language skill develop in the two isolated hemispheres: the right hemisphere showing a deficit, not in the conceptual or semantic features of language, but rather in the 'organisational, analytic, syntactic and hierarchic aspects'.

Summary

At the beginning of this chapter, it was claimed that all research is based on certain assumptions about the nature of the process to be studied; and it was suggested that up to now it has frequently been assumed that language is sequentially organised – despite the large number of recent and compelling arguments to the contrary. Secondly, it was pointed out that any theory concerning an underlying disability must be able to account for the observed behaviour. It was therefore suggested that the hypothesis of a sequential deficit in dysphasic children did not explain adequately many of the observed facts related to their language production. Using current assumptions about the hierarchical organisation of language structure in conjunction with a preliminary study of the writings of dysphasic children, it was concluded that the deficit in these children *may* be some kind of hierarchical structuring disability. This hypothesis received some additional support from observations and studies reporting deficits of rhythmic abilities in these children. There are many questions, as well as objections, that can be raised by this hypothesis – for example, the question of whether the impairment is an inability to deal with hierarchically ordered material, or whether the deficit stems from a basic impairment of rhythm, especially as rhythmic ability has been shown to be a basic element in the comprehension and production of language. A further question raised by this view is whether the deficit extends beyond the inability to deal with hierarchically ordered language structure; that is to say, whether it is specific to language and to rhythm or is present in other types of behaviour. If this latter view is correct, then why is the impairment not displayed in motor or other types of sequential ability? The hypothesis of a hierarchical ordering disability in dysphasic children raises a great number of questions, but by opening up a new direction in research it may well prove to be of service.

Acknowledgements

My thanks are due to Maria Black for her help with the presentation of the puppet show mentioned on pp. 118–120.

References

Barna, S. (1975). Childhood Aphasia: A Preliminary Investigation of Some Auditory and Linguistic Variables. Unpublished Bachelor's thesis, Brunel University.

Benton, A. L. (1964). Developmental aphasia and brain damage. *Cortex* 1, 40–52.

Bever, T. G., Lackner, J. and Kirk, R. (1969). The underlying structure sentence as the primary unit of speech. *Percept. Psychophys.* 5, 225–234.

Bowerman, M. (1973). 'Early Syntactic Development'. Cambridge University Press, Cambridge.

Chomsky, N. (1959). A review of B. F. Skinner's 'Verbal Behaviour'. *Language* 35, 26–58.

Chomsky, N. (1965). 'Aspects of the Theory of Syntax'. M.I.T. Press, Cambridge, Massachusetts.

Chomsky, N. (1976). 'Reflections on Language'. Maurice Temple Smith, Ltd, London.

Critchley, M. (1953). 'The Parietal Lobes'. Edward Arnold and Co, London.

Cromer, R. F. (1974). The Development of Language and Cognition: The Cognition Hypothesis. *In* 'New Perspectives in Child Development' (B. Foss, ed.), pp. 184–252. Penguin Books, Harmondsworth, Middlesex.

Cromer, R. F. (1975). Are Subnormals Linguistic Adults? *In* 'Language Cognitive Deficits and Retardation' (N. O'Connor, ed.), pp. 169–187, Butterworths, London.

Cromer, R. F. (1976). The Cognitive Hypothesis of Language Acquisition and its Implications for Child Language Deficiency. *In* 'Normal and Deficient Child Language' (D. M. Morehead and A. E. Morehead, eds), pp. 283–333. University Park Press, Baltimore.

Day, R. S. (1970). Temporal order perception of a reversible phoneme cluster. Status report on speech research, Haskins Laboratories, *SR* 24, 47–56.

Dennis, M. and Whitaker, H. A. (1976). Language acquisition following hemidecortication: Linguistic superiority of the left over the right hemisphere. *Brain Lang.* 3, 404–433.

Doehring, D. G. (1960). Visual spatial memory in aphasic children. *J. Speech Hear. Res.* 3, 138–149.

Dooling, J. D. (1974). Rhythm and syntax in sentence perception. *J. Verbal Learn. Verbal Behav.* 13, 255–264.

Efron, R. (1963). Temporal perception, aphasia, and déjà vu. *Brain* 86, 403–424.

Eimas, P. D. (1974). Linguistic Processing of Speech by Young Infants. *In* 'Language Perspectives – Acquisition, Retardation, and Intervention' (R. L. Schiefelbusch and L. L. Lloyd, eds), pp. 55–73. University Park Press, Baltimore.

Eisenson, J. (1968). Developmental aphasia: A speculative view with therapeutic implications. *J. Speech Hear. Dis.* 33, 3–13.

Fry, D. B., Abramson, A. S., Eimas, P. D. and Liberman, A. M. (1962). The identification and discrimination of synthetic vowels. *Lang. Speech.* 5, 171–188.

Furth, H. G. (1964). Sequence learning in aphasic and deaf children. *J. Speech Hear. Dis.* 29, 171–177.

Glass, A. V., Gazzaniga, M. S. and Premack, D. (1973). Artificial language training in global aphasics. *Neuropsychologia* 11, 95–103.

Griffiths, P. (1972). 'Developmental Aphasia: An Introduction'. Invalid Children's Aid Association, London.

Hermelin, B. and O'Connor, N. (1973). Ordering in recognition memory after ambiguous initial or recognition displays. *Canad. J. of Psychol.* 27, 191–199.

Hirsch, I. J. (1959). Auditory perception of temporal order. *J. of Acoust. Soc. America* 31, 759–767.

Hughes, J. (1972). Language and Communication: Acquisition of a Non-vocal 'Language' by Previously Languageless Children. Unpublished Bachelor of Technology thesis, Brunel University.

Hughes, J. (1974/75). Acquisition of a non-vocal 'language' by aphasic children. *Cognition* 3, 41–55.

Hughlings-Jackson, J. (1888). On a particular variety of epilepsy ('intellectual aura'), one case with symptoms of organic brain disease. *Brain* 11, 179–207.

Jenkins, J. J. and Palermo, D. S. (1964). Mediation Processes and the Acquisition of Linguistic Structure. *In* 'The Acquisition of Language' (U. Bellugi and R. Brown, eds), Vol. 29, serial no. 92, 141–169. Monographs of the Society for Research in Child Development.

Kracke, I. (1975). Perception of rhythmic sequences by receptive aphasic and deaf children. *Brit. J. of Dis. Comm.* 10, 43–51.

Lashley, K. S. (1951). The Problem of Serial Order in Behaviour. *In* 'Cerebral Mechanisms in Behaviour' (L. A. Jeffress, ed.), pp. 112–136. John Wiley and Sons, Inc., New York.

Lea, J. (1970). 'The Colour Pattern Scheme: A Method of Remedial Language Teaching'. Moor House School, Oxted, Surrey.

Lowe, A. D. and Campbell, R. A. (1965). Temporal discrimination in aphasoid and normal children. *J. Speech Hear. Res.* **8**, 313–314.

Malone, R. L. (1967). Temporal ordering and speech identification abilities. *J. Speech Hear. Res.* **10**, 542–548.

Mark, H. J. and Hardy, W. G. (1958). Orienting reflex disturbances in central auditory or language handicapped children. *J. Speech Hear. Dis.* **23**, 237–242.

Martin, J. G. (1972). Rhythmic (hierarchical) versus serial structure in speech and other behaviour. *Psychol. Rev.* **79**, 487–509.

McReynolds, L. V. (1966). Operant conditioning for investigating speech sound discrimination in aphasic children. *J. Speech Hear. Res.* **9**, 519–528.

Miller, G. A. and Chomsky, N. (1963). Finitary Models of Language Users. *In* 'Handbook of Mathematical Psychology' (R. D. Luce, R. R. Bush and E. Galanter, eds), Vol. II, pp. 419–491. John Wiley and Sons, Inc., New York.

Millikan, C. H. and Darley, F. L. (eds.) (1967). 'Brain Mechanisms Underlying Speech and Language', p. 32. Grune and Stratton, New York and London.

Monsees, E. K. (1961). Aphasia in children. *J. Speech Hear. Dis.* **26**, 83–86.

Myerson, R. and Goodglass, H. (1972). Transformational grammars of three agrammatic patients. *Lang. Speech* **15**, 40–50.

Neisser, U. (1967). 'Cognitive Psychology'. Appleton-Century-Crofts, New York.

O'Connor, N. and Hermelin, B. M. (1973a). Short-term memory for the order of pictures and syllables by deaf and hearing children. *Neuropsychologia* **11**, 437–442.

O'Connor, N. and Hermelin, B. M. (1973b). The spatial or temporal organization of short-term memory. *Quart. J. exp. Psychol.* **25**, 335–343.

Olson, J. L. (1961). Differential diagnosis: Deaf and sensory aphasic children. *Except. Child.* **28**, 422–424.

Perkins, D. N. (1974). Coding position in a sequence by rhythmic grouping. *Mem. Cognition* **2**, 219–223.

Petrie, I. (1975). Characteristics and progress of a group of language disordered children with severe receptive difficulties. *Brit. J. Dis. Comm.* **10**, 123–133.

Poppen, R., Stark, J., Eisenson, J., Forrest, T. and Wertheim, G. (1969). Visual sequencing performance of aphasic children. *J. Speech Hear. Res.* **12**, 288–300.

Premack, D. (1969). A Functional Analysis of Language. Invited address before the American Psychological Association, Washington DC.

Rees, N. S. (1973). Auditory processing factors in language disorders: The view from Procrustes' bed. *J. Speech Hear. Dis.* **38**, 304–315.

Robinson, G. M. and Solomon, D. J. (1974). Rhythm is processed by the speech hemisphere. *J. Exp. Psychol.* **102**, 508–511.

Rosenstein, J. (1957). Tactile perception of rhythmic patterns by normal, blind, deaf, and aphasic children. *Am. Ann. Deaf* **102**, 399–403.

Rosenthal, W. S. (1971). Auditory Threshold-duration Functions in Aphasic Subjects: Implications for the Interaction of Linguistic and Auditory Processing in Aphasia. Paper delivered at the 47th annual convention of the American Speech and Hearing Association, Chicago, Illinois, November.

Rosenthal, W. S. (1972). Auditory and Linguistic Interaction in Developmental Aphasia: Evidence from Two Studies of Auditory Processing. *In* 'Papers and Reports on Child Language Development'. Special Issue: Language Disorders in Children (D. Ingram, ed.), No. 4, pp. 19–34.

Rosenthal, W. S. and Eisenson, J. (1970). Auditory Temporal Order in Aphasic Children as a Function of Selected Stimulus Features. Paper delivered at the 46th annual convention of the American Speech and Hearing Association, New York, November.

Schnitzer, M. L. (1974). Aphasiological evidence for five linguistic hypotheses. *Language* **50**, 300–315.

Sheehan, J. G., Aseltine, S. and Edwards, A. E. (1973). Aphasic comprehension of time spacing. *J. Speech Hear. Res.* **16**, 650–657.

Skinner, B. F. (1957). 'Verbal Behaviour'. Appleton-Century-Crofts, Inc., New York.

Stark, J. (1967). A comparison of the performance of aphasic children on three sequencing tasks. *J. Comm. Dis.* **1**, 31–34.

Stark, J., Poppen, R. and May, M. Z. (1967). Effects of alterations of prosodic features on the sequencing performance of aphasic children. *J. Speech Hear. Res.* **10**, 849–855.

Tallal, P. and Piercy, M. (1973a). Defects of non-verbal auditory perception in children with developmental aphasia. *Nature* 16 February, **241**, 468–469.

Tallal, P. and Piercy, M. (1973b). Developmental aphasia: Impaired rate of non-verbal processing as a function of sensory modality. *Neuropsycholgia* **11**, 389–398.

Tallal, P. and Piercy, M. (1974). Developmental aphasia: Rate of auditory processing and selective impairment of consonant perception. *Neuropsychologia* **12**, 83–93.

Tallal, P. and Piercy, M. (1975). Developmental aphasia: The perception of brief vowels and extended stop consonants. *Neuropsychologia* **13**, 69–74.

Tzortzis, C. and Albert, M. L. (1974). Impairment of memory for sequences in conduction aphasia. *Neuropsychologia* **12**, 355–366.

Wilson, L. F., Doehring, D. G. and Hirsh, I. J. (1960). Auditory discrimination learning by aphasic and nonaphasic children. *J. Speech Hear. Res.* **3**, 130–137.

Withrow, F. B. Jr (1964). Immediate recall by aphasic, deaf and normal children for visual forms presented simultaneously or sequentially. *Asha* **6**, 386.

Worster-Drought, C. and Allen, I. M. (1929). Congenital auditory imperception – Report of a case with congenital word deafness. *J. Neurol. Psychopath.* **9**, 193–208.

Linguistic Problems in Children with Developmental Dysphasia

Paula Menyuk

Introduction

For a long time it was held that children who suffered a language disorder from suspected neurological abnormalities were, except for language, cognitively intact. That is, it was thought that these children's perceptual-motor abilities, as well as thinking and reasoning in the non-linguistic domain, were equal to those of normal children of the same age. Thus the label dysphasic, or aphasic, was applied to these children to emphasise the presence of a specific language disorder. This point of view accords with the notion that the process of language acquisition is unique and that neurophysiological substrates for language processing are specific to verbal tasks. The basis for these assumptions was derived from the performance of aphasic children on standard tests of intelligence. It has been found, in the majority of studies, that on performance (i.e. non-verbal) tests these children attained values equivalent to average or above average intelligence.

While the notion of a specific language disorder was accepted by some workers, other findings suggested that these children had difficulty in processing incoming information which was not confined to the linguistic sphere. For example, it was found that dysphasic children have difficulty in non-linguistic auditory processing (Tallal and Piercy, 1973) and also in visual-motor memory (Levy and Menyuk, 1975). Linguistic and non-linguistic processing abilities are somewhat related in that when the task requirements are similar the degree of difficulty is the same for both verbal and non-verbal tasks. Thus, an aphasic child has difficulty in remembering both a sequence of high and low tones of short duration and consonant-vowel syllables in which information about consonant identification is presented for comparatively short periods of time. On the other hand the aphasic child can succeed with tones of longer duration as well as steady-state vowels. This suggests that increased *exposure* to acoustic information is necessary whether the nature of the information is linguistic or non-linguistic. Similarly, aphasic children have difficulty in repeating a motor task presented visually and involving more than one actor, action and object relation. They also have difficulty in acting out these relations when the information is given acoustically, in sentence form. They can, however, carry out both tasks when the relations are limited.

The above findings suggest that the processing abilities necessary to identify the properties of categories (i.e. whether they are speech or non-speech categories), and to recall the relations between categories (i.e. specific relations between actors, actions and objects), are somehow impaired in these children. However, no relation of dependency between *acquisitions* in either domain is implied. Many of the studies examining cognitive and linguistic development, both in normal children and aphasic children, are unable to show clearly relations of dependency between such acquisitions (Menyuk, 1975a, b). If, however, the above findings showing difficulties in processing non-linguistic as well as linguistic material are correct, then it is difficult to understand why these children have been found to perform within the average or above average range on non-verbal aspects of intelligence tests. One might conclude that this contradiction is due to the inadequacy of standard psychometric tests; that is, they do not sample the appropriate abilities, or else do not distinguish clearly between linguistic and non-linguistic tasks.

Although both of the above explanations seem feasible, alternative interpretations could be advanced. First there is a possibility of marked differences in processing abilities within the dysphasic group. But these differences are masked when only mean values for the group are presented. Secondly it is possible that the differences in processing ability only apply to the sphere of language. These differences manifest themselves as specific difficulties with the input or output processing of the phonological, morphological, syntactic or semantic components of language. But since these components are inter-related, a more reasonable notion is that the underlying processing difficulty affects one or more of the components of language, depending upon the nature of the task. The posited relations between language components are represented graphically in Fig. 1.

On the basis of the above arguments the contents of this chapter will rest on the following assumptions:

1 Certain processing difficulties underlie the language impairment of aphasic children, and the same difficulties may also underlie deficits in their non-linguistic behaviour.

2 There are differences in linguistic and non-linguistic processing

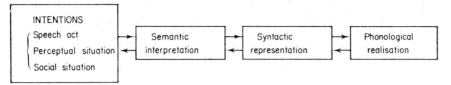

Fig. 1. Development of M.M.U. (mean morphemes per utterance) with age in a normally developing population and a language disordered population.

abilities among dysphasic children as well as between dysphasic and normal children.

The pages that follow will be devoted to reviewing the findings of studies which have either analysed the spontaneous language production of aphasic children or else have sampled their language behaviour in experimental situations. The available material covering these aspects of language is, however, very limited.

The chapter will also attempt to provide explanations for the behaviour observed.

Studies based on Spontaneous Language Behaviour

The primary purpose of studies of the spontaneous language behaviour of dysphasic children has largely been directed to examining, in much greater detail than by use of any existing standardised test, possible differences between the language production of dysphasic and that of normal children. The language behaviour of aphasic children has been sampled in varying contextual situations. The usual procedure is to engage the child in conversation with the experimenter, making a record of the language and then analysing the sample obtained. Most of these studies are horizontal in nature; that is, one sample is obtained from each child. The variables that are usually examined are the structures produced and the age at which these structures are produced. Comparisons are then made between the structures produced by dysphasic children and those from normal children of the same age or younger. Different ways of eliciting verbal output have been used, for instance responses given to pictures or real objects, free conversations with no specific stimuli present, and language directed to others as well as to the experimenter. Different constraints have been placed on what is to be considered a language sample. Some experimenters have imposed a number constraint by analysing, for example, the first 50, the mid-50, or 100 utterances; others have used a time constraint (30 minutes or one hour of speech sampling);

and still others a stimulus situation constraint (when all the pictures or objects have been discussed). Longhurst and Schrandt (1973) have attempted a comparison of four procedures in the analysis of aphasic children's speech. It is clear that, given all the variations in language sampling, one should be cautious in generalising about the results of these studies. Moreover, many of the children investigated have been in a therapeutic situation, which might have resulted in their language being, at least in part, a product not of their own generalisations but of those supplied by the therapists.

The findings of the above studies can be summarised as follows: First, the types of sentences produced by the dysphasic children are similar to those produced by normal children; however, sentence structure in the dysphasic group is representative of that produced by younger children (Morehead and Ingram, 1973). Secondly, there are significant differences between the dysphasic and non-dysphasic groups in the frequency with which certain structures are produced. The dysphasic children produce well-formed sentence types less frequently than do normal children, and conversely produce poorly formed structures (approximations to well-formed sentences) more frequently than normal children (Leonard, 1972). One might conclude from these results that dysphasic children show a delay in language development which varies in degree of severity, and that their language development, in terms of sentence structure, approximates to that of normal younger children. Since most of the language samples in the dysphasic group have been obtained from children 3 years of age and older, it is difficult to establish the pattern of *early* language development. But on the basis of the findings suggesting that these children's language production is simply delayed one could assume that in terms of *sequence* of acquisition of sentence forms the two groups (normal and dysphasic) follow a parallel course.

A second view of the language behaviour of dysphasic children is that the pattern of their language development differs from that of normal children in two ways. Firstly, some aspects of language will *remain* unchanged in the dysphasic children unless a concentrated effort is made to help development (Lee, 1966); and, secondly, there are particular aspects of the language which are extremely difficult for these children to acquire, and thus plateaus in development are likely to occur (Menyuk, 1964). In summary, this second view holds that there is no time when the language development of the dysphasic merely matches that of a younger normal child.

Morehead and Ingram (1973) compared the structure of the utterances produced by 15 normal and 15 aphasic children who were at approximately the same stage of M.M.U. (mean morphemes per utterance). The sample size used for analysis ranged from 80 to 200 utterances. The language samples were collected in a free play situation with the experimenter or parent, whilst the children played with toys and looked at a book. It was found that there were few significant differences in the syntactic structures used by the two groups at equivalent stages of M.M.U. The development of phrase structure was similar and, of the 40 transformations compared, only 4 were significantly more frequent in the language sample of the normal children (question with auxiliary, do segment, locative, demonstrative and noun deletion), while 2 were more frequent in the sample of the aphasic group (progressive affix and plural affix). This latter finding may be related to the great emphasis placed on the development of morphological rules of tense and number in most teaching programmes for aphasic children. Morehead and Ingram also found that significant differences between the two groups were seen both in the frequency with which transformations occur and in the use of the question form. In addition there were significant differences in the number of major lexical categories (noun, main verb, copula, adjective) used for each type of construction. An examination of the list of construction types identified by the experimenters in the language samples indicated that, at the first level of M.M.U. (2 +), 14 types are used by the normal children and 13 are used by the aphasic children, whereas at M.M.U. 5 + (the last level sampled) 43 are used by the normal and 31 by the aphasic children. At the first level 8 of the constructions used overlap, whilst at the last level overlap was seen in 22 constructions. The primary distinction between the two groups appears to be in the number of different question forms used and also the use of conjunctions and different relative clause and complement forms. This seems to be in keeping with the finding concerning use of transformations; that is, transformations which are normally infrequently used are even less common among aphasic children. In summary, the experimenters found that there were significant differences in the frequency of use of certain syntactic structures and in the number of major lexical categories used per construction type. Moreover, these findings seem to be inextricably confounded. The experimenters, however, suggest a *representational* deficit to account for the differences found. Morehead and Ingram state that the utterances produced by the aphasic children were, on the whole, less well-formed than those of the normal children.

The findings of this study also indicate that there are significant differences in the *rate* at which different sentence types are acquired by the two groups and, therefore, in the rate at which M.M.U. increases. That is to say, the gap between the two groups, in terms of different constructions used, widens with time. It is only at the very early stages of development of M.M.U. (i.e. 2 +) that the use of constructions is only slightly different. The results concerning M.M.U. indicate that there is a direct relationship between length of structures (if not their complexity) and the time taken to acquire them. That is to say, longer structures take longer to acquire. Figure 2 presents the data of the study of Morehead and Ingram concerning M.M.U., showing the comparative ages for achieving M.M.U. 2+ (the first level) and M.M.U. 5+ (the last level) for both groups. The age differences at the intermediate M.M.U. levels are based upon the assumption of a linear increase in utterance length; the end points, however, are based on actual data and clearly indicates a widening gap.

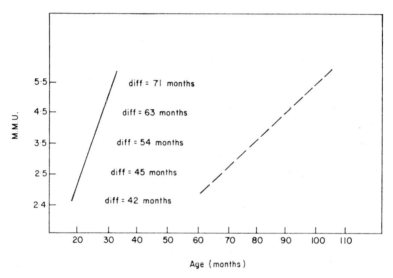

Age (months)

Fig. 2. A graphic representation of relations between components in the language. (M.M.U., mean morphemes per utterance; – – –, dysphasic children; ——, normal children.)

Menyuk (1964) collected language samples from 10 children in preschool and kindergarten classes who were said to use 'infantile' speech, and 10 children with normal language development. The two groups were matched for age, IQ (a vocabulary test), sex and socio-economic status. The mean sample size used for analysis was 74 and 80 utterances respectively. The children's age ranged from 3 years to 5 years 2 months. None of the children were receiving therapy for their 'infantile' speech. Language was sampled in three stimulus situations: description of pictures, conversation with the experimenter using a set list of questions for each child, and a role-playing group situation in which the children were pretending to be a family. The results of the analysis disclosed two main points: firstly that only few of the children labelled as 'infantile' used the *range* of structures of normal speaking children, and secondly that most of the significant differences in the use of structures involved permutations within sentences (e.g. 'there' and 'do' insertion) or else elaboration (e.g. conjunction and relative clause). More of the children with 'infantile' speech used non-grammatical forms (or approximations to well-formed sentences) and used them significantly more frequently than the normal speaking children. Most of the approximations of the 'infantile' group consisted of omissions in a sentence (noun phrase, verb phrase, preposition, article, markers of tense) whereas the normal speaking group, for the most part, used alternate forms (or substitutions) rather than omissions. Furthermore, whilst in the group of children speaking normally there was a significant correlation between age and reduction in the use of approximate forms, no such correlation was demonstrated in the group with 'infantile' speech.

One other comparison was made in this study. A language sample of a 3-year-old in the 'infantile' group was compared with several samples collected from a child with normal language development tested over one whole year, i.e. from the age of 2 to the age of 3. The purpose of this comparison was to observe whether or not the 3-year-old child with 'infantile' speech was using structures similar to those used by the 2-year-old with normal language development. It was found that the language used by the 3-year-old – with infantile speech – was more sophisticated both in terms of base structure rules and transformations. The normal child, however, at 3 years of age was using transformational structures, which were only present in the speech of less than 50 per cent of the children in the 'infantile' group over the entire age range. These involved either permutation (as in the case of the passive construction) or sentence elaboration (as in conjunction and embedding). In addition, many of the approximations to well-formed sentences found in the language sample of the normally speaking 2-year-old (primarily those of omission) were used by the children over the older age range of the 'infantile' group, whereas by age 3 the normal child and other children with normal speech development were using substitutions of classes. The experimenter concluded that the term 'infantile' seemed to be a misnomer, since at no age level did the grammatical production of a child with such 'infantile' speech match that of a normally developing child. Furthermore, there were only a few instances, over the age range of the 'infantile' speech group, of both the use of various well-formed structures and the reduction of use of approximate forms. Thus, little 'catching up' was going on in this group. In other words, a plateau in language development appeared to have been reached by the language disordered children.

Lee (1966) compared the sentence types used in 'spontaneous speech' by a normal child aged 3 years 1 month and a language disordered child of 4 years 7 months. The analysis of the language samples led Lee to conclude that there were differences both in the structure and in the frequency with which utterances were produced. The utterances of the language disordered child were frequently without a subject. Most of the utterances consisted of *verb phrases* with object alone ('go school', 'eat supper', etc.), with prepositional phrases ('do with hand') or with an additional verb phrase ('want wake up'). Some utterances were simply concatenations of subjects, verbs and objects ('Linda, Debbie, sick, listen, radio.'). It should be noted that these utterances mark the *main* predicate relations of verb + object (or prepositional phrase, or sentence), and in some instances (as in the concatenated example given above) subject + predicate relations are in an appropriate *order*, but there is little else of sentence structure. In context they are nevertheless, interpretable utterances. This was also true of the utterances obtained from the 'infantile' group in the study cited above. Lee concluded that the language disordered child was not merely slower in following a normal pattern of development but was failing to produce certain types of syntactic structures.

Lee (1974) has since developed a method of scoring and analysing language samples obtained from language disordered children. Although there is not a summary of the data obtained from the language disordered children, she discusses two cases in detail (see pp. 176–94) which shed some light on comparative patterns of development. Lee compared a normal child aged 2 years 1 month and a language disordered child of 3 years 7 months. The findings, using the sentence scoring technique, indicated that the language disordered child was approximately at the language development level of a normal 23-month-old child. Lee further states that the language behaviour of the normal child and that of the language disordered child were quite similar. On the other hand, when comparisons were made on the use of structures marked differences were present. The child with a language problem seemed more advanced than the normal in some aspects but less advanced in others. For example, the language disordered child modified nouns by a greater range of attributive terms (size, colour, possessive pronoun, and number), and verbs by a greater range of locative particles (down, off, back) than the normal child; she also expanded the noun phrase with *two* terms ('That little car . . .'). There were, however, a number of structures present in the normal child's sample that were not found in the sample of the child with language problems. These structures were noun plural markers, articles, verb tense markers, possessive markers, copula, auxiliary *be* and modal *can*. An analysis of the mean length of utterance of the two children's language sample indicated that it was approximately the same (3·6 for the deviant speaking child and 3·5 for the normal speaking child). Thus while these two children were at approximately the *same* level of language development by two scoring techniques (sentence scoring and mean length of utterance) the structures they used varied.

Leonard (1972) compared the language of 9 normal speaking and 9 'defective' speaking children matched for age (mean 5 years 3 months), scores on the Peabody Picture Vocabulary Test and socio-economic status. He analysed a language sample of 50 utterances, obtained by asking the children to relate a story about pictures. Comparisons were then made of the frequency with which various structures were used. Significant differences were found between the two groups in the frequency with which they used 14 structures, some of which were well formed and others approximations. The structures more frequently used by the normal children were conjunction and embedding (infinitival complements with and without objects such as 'I want to go'. and 'I want him to go'.), contraction of copula (this might be accounted for by greater frequency of omission of copula in the language disordered group), pronoun forms, the auxiliary 'be', adjective, and negation. The approximations more frequently used by the language disordered group were article, noun phrase and verb phrase omission, and verb number constraint in 'there' insertion, for instance 'There's the bears'.

The results of the studies of the spontaneous language production of children with language problems (which might, indeed, vary from one group to another) can be summarised as follows: (a) Language-retarded children are, on the whole, delayed in the sentence types they produce and this delay becomes more marked with increasing age, as the normally developing child begins to acquire the specific rules of the language approximately when he is 2½ years old; (b) Language disordered children are *particularly delayed* in acquiring structures which involve permutations of major categories within the sentence (as in negative and question) or elaboration of basic relations, by expanding the noun phrase or verb phrase of the sentence using other major syntactic categories (article, auxiliary and modal verbs), or elaboration of the sentence as in conjunction and embedding; and (c) approximations to *well*-formed structures are significantly more frequent and they persist over a fairly long period of development.

The findings about semantic development are equivocal. It is not clear whether this aspect of language development shows deficits comparable to those of structural development. Semantic development seems to be more advanced than structural development in the language retarded children, because they preserve in their verbal utterances, to a great extent, the *main relations* of actor, action and object. Semantic development can be interpreted, however, as lexical acquisition (i.e. the comprehension of properties of words) and acquisition of relations (i.e. comprehension of actor, action, object, coordinate and subordinate relations in utterances). The performance of language disordered children on standard vocabulary tests indicates retardation, although there are exceptions, for instance the findings reported by Menyuk (1964) and Leonard (1972). Such studies, however, provide little information about the particular semantic fields (nominal, verbal, attributive) and especially those with which these children have difficulty in spontaneous speech production (e.g. locative and temporal terms). Although it has often been reported that they have difficulty with, for example, spatial terms in tests of comprehension, it is not clear whether the same difficulty exists in their spontaneous language.

Morehead and Ingram (1973) have suggested that a semantic deficit might be the cause of the structural deficit. That is, when the child begins to understand structural relations between objects and events in the environment he also relates the events to the language which is used to encode them; and when new lexical items are acquired new structural expressions are needed to fit their relationships. For example, when the child acquires *different* verb categories (those that take simple objects *and* those that take complement structures) he expands the structures that can serve as objects to these verb categories (Limber, 1973).

Language production requires knowledge of semantic relations; in turn syntactic forms are needed to express these relations and phonological categories and rules are required to realise them. All the language disordered children appear to have difficulty with the phonological aspects of language, although the nature of the difficulty varies from child to child. Some of these children exhibit arrested development for long periods of time, but, nevertheless, appear to follow the sequence of phonological distinctions observed with normal children, while others appear to evolve unique realisation rules (Menyuk, 1968). One point of interest in these children is the degree to which they maintain the features of the target speech sequences. For example, if the target sound is initial $/\theta/$, and it is realised as either $/f/$ or $/t/$, there is little change in feature composition of the sound. If, however, it is realised as $/b/$ or $/\phi/$ then there is a large difference. Also of interest is the question of the variability in the speech sound realisation rules, that is to say, how stable is the production from time to time and across time, as well as the effect of context on realisation rules. All of these factors play a role in normal phonological development and presumably also in defective language development. Although there is a great deal of data on the performance of language disordered children on standard tests, adequate information as to their phonological development in spontaneous speech is not available. A few observations, however, indicate either a general retardation or else a set of specific problems, but no information on the factors discussed above is available. In addition, most experimenters limit the sampling of spontaneous speech to the production or imitation of words in isolation (for example, Farwell, 1972).

Studies based on Experimental Situations

Most experimental studies on children with developmental dysphasia have been attempts to assess both their linguistic and non-linguistic behaviours by using a variety of tests designed to sample a wide range of cognitive functions thought to be relevant to their specific difficulties. For example, Weiner (1972) assessed 8 dysphasic boys with a variety of tests and re-tested 7 of these children a year later. He compared their performance with that of 7 normal boys matched for age, IQ (which was in the normal range) and socio-economic status (the experimental group's socio-economic status was somewhat higher than that of the control group). The tests examined auditory discrimination, grammatical comprehension, auditory-vocal abilities (repetition of words and sentences and an articulation test) and oral-motor abilities (examination of diadochokinetic abilities). Weiner also examined visual perceptual abilities such as figure-ground discrimination and performance on visual sequencing tasks, together with the Bender-Gestalt and Harris draw-a-man and -woman tests. The results in the dysphasic group in the first and second assessment were virtually identical. They had difficulty in articulation but not in *sequencing*. The results on the material which had been presented orally showed significant differences when compared with the performance of the normal children, but none of the tasks presented visually showed significant differences. Comprehension of grammatical structures in the 2 groups was also significantly different. In addition, the dysphasic children showed a significantly poorer performance on auditory-vocal abilities, oral-motor abilities, and the scores of the Bender-Gestalt and 'draw-a-person' tests. It is important to note that the dysphasic children exhibited no difficulty in *sequencing* abilities either in linguistic or non-linguistic tasks in the auditory-vocal, motor or visual modalities. Weiner concluded that the dysphasic children have attentional and perceptual problems, along with difficulties in the organisation of motor patterns and also in dealing with verbal symbols. These results are analogous to those found in a number of other studies in similar groups of dysphasic children. But despite the agreement of results, two questions remain unanswered: First, what are the exact processing difficulties which embrace all the tests in which the dysphasic children fail, and, second, do *all* the dysphasic children have *all* these problems?

Several studies have examined the ability of dysphasic children to repeat (immediately recall) linguistic material of varied structure. For example Menyuk (1964) examined children with 'infantile' speech patterns. The children were asked to repeat grammatical and non-grammatical

sentences representing sentence types produced by normal children between the ages of 2 years 1 month and 7 years 1 month. Their ability to
repeat was compared to that of a matched group of normal children and
to their own ability to produce spontaneously various sentence types. The
results disclosed several findings of interest: (*a*) The language disordered
children made considerable numbers of omissions, leaving out whole
sentences or phrases in conjoined and embedded sentences; (*b*) the dysphasic children were unable to repeat successfully some of the structures
that they were able to produce spontaneously; (*c*) approximations to complete repetitions remained the same throughout the age range (3 years to
5 years 1 month); and (*d*) in the language disordered children – but not
the normal children – sentence length correlated significantly with the
accuracy of repetition. In general, the ability to repeat sentences seemed
to be quite analogous to that of their spontaneous speech, the only
exception being that they could not repeat some structures which they
could produce in spontaneous speech. The inverse occurred with the
normal children, in that they were able to repeat structures that were not
present in their spontaneous speech. The findings were thought to indicate
the presence of a short-term memory deficit in the language disordered
children.

The results of the above study were equivocal over the question of
whether the length *or* the structure of the sentence affected repetition,
since these two factors were confounded in the types of sentence used in
the study. Furthermore, the effect of meaningfulness of the phonological
sequences on its subsequent recall was not examined, since all the material
used in this test was meaningful. One might speculate that the behaviour
being examined was in fact the ability of language disordered children to
echo the sentences rather than the ability to process linguistic material.
Such a possibility, however, seems doubtful, since the systematic modifications which reflected levels of structural development found in their
spontaneous speech occur in both groups. These questions were pursued
in a further study (Menyuk and Looney, 1972a, b) which examined both
language disordered and normal children in their ability to repeat various
sentences (active-declarative, imperative, negative and question) of 3–5
words in length – 5 words being the upper limit for these children. The
children were also tested with a set of active-declarative sentences containing, in varying positions, American-English singleton and cluster
phonological categories, and a set of 3 nonsense syllables in which the
manner or place of articulation was varied. The two groups were approximately matched on the basis of their performance in the Peabody
Picture Vocabulary Test (dysphasic group, 6 years 1 month; normal
group, 5 years 11 months), but the mean age of the two groups varied
(dysphasic group, 6 years 4 months; normal group, 4 years 7 months).

The language disordered children were drawn from a speech clinic, and all were receiving therapy.

The results of this study indicated marked differences in their ability to repeat between the two groups. Of interest was the finding that given sentence lengths of 3–5 words the performance of the language disordered group was more significantly affected by *structure* than by length (3-word-long sentences were accurately repeated by most of these children). On the other hand, the normal children showed no difference in the ability to repeat sentences varying either in length or in structure. Language disordered children fell into two different groups – those who omitted the auxiliary/modal aspects of the negative and question sentences, and those who repeated these aspects but did not apply the appropriate transformational operations. For example, the first group of children would repeat sentences such as 'He can't go home' as 'He no go (home)' and 'Where does he go?' as 'Where he go?', while the second group repeated these sentences as 'He no can go' and 'Where he do go?'. It is important, however, to notice that the meaning-bearing elements of sentence intention (negation or question) and relations (subject and predicate) are maintained in both types of repetition. This is quite analogous to the behaviour observed in spontaneous sentence production. The meaningfulness of the stimuli presented affected the accuracy of repetition. Both normal speaking and language disordered children repeated the phonological sequences more accurately in words than in nonsense syllables. Further evidence of the effect of meaningfulness on recall for the language disordered children was that final singletons or clusters which marked number or tense were often omitted, except when they were part of the word stem. For example 'bees' might be repeated as 'bee', but 'nose' was never repeated as 'no'. Thus one might assume that a lexical 'look-up' procedure (i.e. a scanning of the dictionary available to the child using both basic syntactic and semantic information) was used in their recall rather than a simple categorisation of phonological segments. The degree of meaningfulness was also found to affect the performance of the language disordered children in another study designed to examine their ability to process speech and non-speech acoustic information. Thus, Rosenthal (1972) found that language disordered as well as normal children processed speech stimuli more successfully than non-speech stimuli.

Distinctive feature composition of the words and nonsense-syllables used for recall in the experiments of Menyuk and Looney (1972a, b) affected accuracy of repetition and both groups showed somewhat similar difficulties, although to differing degrees, in feature maintenance of the target consonantal stimuli. Thus both groups tended in their substitutions to maintain the features of $\pm$ nasal, $\pm$ obstruant and $\pm$ consonantal to a greater degree than the features of $\pm$ voice, $\pm$ strident, $\pm$ continuant (manner features) and ± anterior, and ± coronal (place features). There was a significant correlation between the number of errors made in repetition of syntactic structures and phonological sequences by the language disordered children. That is, those children who had the most difficulty in processing and reproducing the particular structural aspects of the sentence also had the greatest difficulty in processing and re-producing the speech sound segments of words in sentences.

In summary, the above experiments seem to show that there is a hierarchical organisation in the processing of information reflected in the immediate recall of sentences. Language disordered children preserve best the intention of the sentence (to command, declare, negate and question) and the main relations in the sentence (actor-action and frequently object). They also preserve the syntactic rule of *word order* to express this relation. They do not, however, preserve the transformational modifications used to express the intention and relations in the sentence, and the specific phonological segments of the speech signal. There was a significant cor-relation between individual performances in the ability to preserve the structural and the phonological aspects of the sentences. A lexical 'look-up procedure' was employed by language disordered children, shown by their ability to distinguish between final segments and clusters which are part of the word stem and those which are added to the stem to mark tense and plural, and also by their greater accuracy in the recall of words as compared to nonsense syllables. These results indicate a much firmer knowledge of lexical items and basic semantic relations than of syntactic and phonological categories and rules used to express these relations. Finally, the differences in performance among the language disordered children did not correlate with age. Given sentence lengths of 3–5 words and a limited set of structures some of the language disordered children used the stimuli presented to repeat aspects of the sentence (auxiliary and modal) not normally present in their spontaneous utterances, while other children did not follow this pattern of response. The first group also made fewer errors in repetition of phonological sequences. Therefore by using sentence repetition a dis-tinction appeared between the language disordered children which was not apparent in the studies of their spontaneous utterances.

Since a significant correlation between syntactic and phonological errors was found in the above cited study one might presume – especially in the case of those children who primarily omitted lexical and phono-logical aspects of the utterances presented – that they were simply not at-tending to all the relevant phonological sequences in the sentence. Furthermore, whether they were hearing the speech signal in a distorted manner or only reproducing it as such was not clear. Although it is difficult to explain the overall behaviour of these children as one of in-attention, some data have shown that placing stress on the first word of a

3-word utterance helps recall not only of the first word but also of the two other items (Stark *et al.*, 1967). This might be interpreted as being indicative of these children's inability to attend to all relevant aspects of the speech signal.

To examine the question of whether lack of attention to relevant acoustic phonological information, or insufficient analysis of it, would account for the repetition performance of these children, and also whether or not the problem was related to their ability to perceive as well as to reproduce the sentences, a study was carried out designed to examine speech sound categorisation abilities in a perception and reproduction task (Menyuk and Looney, In preparation). The task required distinction of place features within speech sound sets. Children were asked to distinguish between /p/, /t/ and /k/; /w/, /r/ and /l/; /b/, /d/ and /g/; and /s/, /t/ and /š/ when only the initial segment varied in a word sequence (for example seat, feet and sheet), and to reproduce these distinctions. All stimuli were recorded and all were equally stressed. Twenty-seven language disordered children between 4 years 1 month and 10 years 10 months of age (mean age 6 years 4 months) and the 19 normal children between 3 years 5 months and 5 years 4 months (mean age 4 years 2 months) were studied. None of the children, language disordered or normal, showed random performances, and patterns of responses emerged in terms of distinctive feature maintenance, indicating that the children were *attending* to relevant acoustic phonological cues. Ample time was allowed for responding (5 s between stimuli) and none of the children appeared to be confused by the task. Patterns of response, in terms of errors, emerged showing differences in processing techniques within the language disordered group, as well as between the normal and the dysphasic children.

Three different patterns of phonological processing (A, B, C,) appeared in the dysphasic children. These differences were related to the percentage of errors in the reproduction as against the percentage of errors in the perception task. There were also differences between children in the specific sets of speech sounds in which there occurred a greater or lesser percentage of errors. The mean percentage of errors for each of the 3 sub-groups (A, B, C,) found within the dysphasic children and the mean percentage of errors made by the normal children are shown in Table 1. Also shown is the rank order of difficulty of each set of speech sounds for each of the sub-groups. This shows that the normal children achieved a better overall performance than any sub-group of the dysphasic children, except for the A group, in the perception task. There were two groups of children whose mean error rates in the perception task exceeded those in the reproduction task (the normal, and C sub-group in the language disordered children), and two in which the inverse occurred (the A and B dysphasic groups). In the A group the children had significantly greater difficulty in the reproduction task than in the perception task, whereas the children in the B group had marked difficulties in both. The rank order of increasing difficulty in perceiving and reproducing elements of the various speech sound sets was quite similar in the normal and dysphasic C groups but different from the A and B groups, which in turn differed from each other.

Table 1

Mean per cent of error in categorising members of speech sound sets and rank order of difficulty among sets

Perception				Production			
Mean % of Error							
Groups				*Groups*			
A	B	C	Normal	A	B	C	Normal
9·2	16·5	18·2	12·6	20·1	24·3	16·7	6·6

Rank Order of Difficulty Among Speech Sound Sets

Groups	*Sets*	*Groups*	*Sets*
A–	sfš <wrl <bdg <ptk	A–	bdg <ptk <wrl <sfš
B–	wrl <sfš <ptk <bdg	B–	ptk <bdg <wrl <sfš
C–	sfš <bdg <wrl <ptk	C–	ptk <sfš <bdg <wrl
Normal–	sfš <bdg <wrl <ptk	Normal–	sfš <ptk <bdg <wrl

The C group of dysphasic children appeared to be the group which can benefit most from the stimuli in a repetition task as can normal children. The children in the A group were unable to overcome their phonological expressive problem despite an immediately present model, and group B had marked difficulty in both tasks. This preliminary study suggests that, if there were significant relations between phonological and structural processing in comprehension and production tasks, then different patterns of processing by the above three groups of children should have been observed when examining these aspects (i.e. phonological and structural) simultaneously. Furthermore, one might expect to observe different patterns of language development in a longitudinal study of these children, but such a study has not yet been carried out.

Although the repetition technique is potentially rewarding in the assessment of language behaviour of dysphasic children, since their responses are not simply echoic but do reflect processing of the input data, it is on the other hand limited by the fact that the exact source of difficulty cannot be determined. In theory the problem encountered by dysphasic children in immediate memory tasks might be one of analysis, comparison or retrieval. Furthermore, the technique does not assess the abilities of dysphasic children to comprehend or spontaneously generate language.

Theoretically the relation between repetition and comprehension and production abilities in normal children is as follows: comprehension < repetition < production. With dysphasic children the relation between production and repetition is clearly quite different. The data indicate the following: Production < repetition. A study was, therefore, undertaken to examine the language processing abilities of these children under varying task requirements. Language behaviour was sampled across six experimental tasks which are frequently used in tests or experimental studies of linguistic competence. These tasks were: (1) Comprehension of structures, assessed by manipulation of toy objects and picture identification; (2) Modelled production, assessed by repetition of structures and correction of non-grammatical structures; (3) Spontaneous generation, assessed by obtaining a sample of 'free' speech and the description of particular pictures. Each task, with the exception of spontaneous speech, contained tokens of the same structures in order that comparisons of structure processing could be made across tasks. Eight principle types of structure which previous research had indicated to be potential sources of difficulty for these children were examined: (1) simple sentences with transitive, intransitive and copular verbs; (2), (3) simple sentences with noun phrase or verb phrase expansion; (4), (5) negative and question sentences; (6), (7) complement and relative clause sentences; and (8) coordinate sentences.

Twenty children, ranging in age from 4 years 8 months to 8 years 2 months, were examined. All of these children were attending hospital, as it was thought that their language difficulties might be related to neurological abnormalities. Fifteen had been diagnosed as having both receptive and expressive language problems, four as having only an expressive problem, and one was diagnosed as a case of delayed language development. Three of the children with receptive and expressive language problems were also described as having 'word-finding' difficulties. A preliminary analysis of this latter group indicates that such a label might cover two distinct groups: those who have a motor planning problem and those who have a lexical 'look-up' problem (Menyuk and Looney, In preparation). All of the children were described as having gross and/or fine motor problems. A preliminary study of normal children indicates that there might be a significant correlation between gross motor skills and verbal output, and between fine motor skills and verbal 'sophistication' (Wolff and Wolff, 1972).

Responses were scored in terms of: (a) sentence hits (full relations in sentences given); (b) morpheme hits (number of separable morphemes encoded or decoded); (c) semantic relations; and (d) fully well formed responses regardless of accuracy (as for example substitution of 'a' for 'the'). All the above types of scoring allowed comparison across tasks, since a child could achieve a 'correct' score in the comprehension tasks (manipulation and identification) without fully analysing the sentence in terms of all function words.

A preliminary analysis of the data indicated that, in general, subjects performed better on the identification and manipulation tasks than on the production and free speech tasks, which in turn were performed better than the repetition and correction tasks. Using the 'sentence hit' scoring method it was found that the order of difficulty in encoding and decoding structures was, in most cases, as follows: simple sentences < negative and question sentences; expansion of noun phrase sentences < expansion of verb phrase sentences; coordinate sentences < relative clause and complement sentences. The above results could have been predicted from previous research. Table 2 indicates the mean scores of subjects in the various tasks and a comparison of the results using two scoring methods on two production tasks. The dysphasic children, as has been found previously, preserve the semantic relations in a sentence much more accurately than they do the particular syntactic forms used to express modifications of these relations (such as determiners, markers of tense, etc.).

Table 2

Mean scores obtained in varying tests of linguistic processing

Tests	Sentence hit score	Semantic relations score
Identification	17·65	
Free Speech	12·30	
Manipulation	10·80	
Repetition	7·40	23·3
Generation	7·05	
Correction	5·05	16·5

These mean scores, however, obscure differences within this group. The data indicate that there was consistency of behaviour *within* tasks (i.e. those who did well on some items within a task tended to do well across items, and conversely) but inconsistency of behaviour *across* tasks (i.e. those who did well on some tasks did not necessarily do well on all of them). On the whole, neither age nor type of dysphasia were good predictors of performance. There was a bimodal distribution in the performance on all tasks; that is to say, one group did comparatively well and another group did comparatively badly. These groups, however, were never identical across tasks. There was one small group of children (4 in number) who appeared to perform consistently worse than the others on the production tasks; however, they did not belong to the same diagnostic group, and the consistently poor performance did not appear in all tasks.

The salient finding disclosed by the experimental studies of the language processing abilities of children who have been labelled dysphasic or simply language disordered is the clear and distinct differences that exist among these children themselves. These differences cannot be simply described as 'degree of deficit', although the actual outcome of the defective processing might appear as a simple delay of language development varying only in degree. There are particular aspects of language with which they have more or less difficulty, but it is not clear that the *same* processing difficulties can account for the *same* product difficulties. There have been a number of descriptions of these processing difficulties, none of which seems totally satisfactory, most probably *because* of the differences discussed above, that exist among children with developmental dysphasia.

Explanations for Language Behaviour

Rees (1973) has openly stated that explanations for the language and learning difficulties in children with developmental dysphasia on the basis of a disorder of auditory-temporal sequencing appear to be unsupported by research findings. Instead, Rees postulates a deficit in cognitive function. Some recent findings, cited previously, indicate that children with developmental dysphasia do not necessarily have a problem in auditory-temporal *sequencing*, but, rather, they have difficulty first in making speech sound distinctions that require temporal judgments (Rosenthal, 1972), and secondly making distinctions between and remembering sequences of auditory events when a *chunk* of that event is of too short a duration (Tallal and Piercy, 1973, 1974). Further, it is clear that differences in the processing of linguistic auditory information and non-linguistic auditory information exist, and at an early age. There are now many reports in the literature suggesting that speech information is channelled and analysed in a different manner from non-speech information, and that these differences in processing exist when the child is only one month old (Eimas, 1974). Finally, it is not clear what Rees means by a 'cognitive deficit', since cognitive development itself is composed of the gradual organisation and integration of different kinds of information.

At least two factors need to be considered in trying to determine the basis of the language difficulty in children with developmental dysphasia. The first is the possibility of variation within the group of children labelled as developmental dysphasia, and we have tried to indicate that both patterns of language development and also on-line processing of language categories and relations may differ between these children. Differences in language behaviour may, in turn, be accounted for by differences in the way in which input information is analysed and stored and/or the way this information is retrieved in output programming. The second factor is the possibility that, with time, changes in normal children occur in both linguistic and non-linguistic processing, and presumably these same changes also occur with language deviant children, although these are likely to be more slow because of their processing difficulties.

We shall examine the last factor first. If one were to plot very roughly changes that occur with time in the normal development of language processing, they would appear to be based upon those aspects of language attended to, analysed and stored, and also on the amount of information and the process by which this information is analysed and stored (Menyuk, 1977). During the first year of life the normal infant is sensitive to both segmental and supra-segmental differences in the speech signal and he makes communicative interaction with his environment (i.e. conveys intentions with babbled utterances). At about the beginning of the second year of life the child develops the ability not only to produce speech signals which express intentions (stating, demanding, requesting, etc.), but also statements about objects and events in his environment. At about 18 months of age the child develops the ability to express relations between objects and events in the environment. At about 24 months of life the full relations of subject and predicate are expressed and the child begins to produce utterances in accordance with the specific rules of the language in his environment. Thus during the first 2–3 years of life there are distinct changes in the ability of a child to attend to his environment, and also in what he selects for encoding. In addition all children imitate during this period, although the amount of echoic behaviour in which they engage varies among different children. This imitative behaviour is an overt testing of the child's hypotheses concerning the categories and re-lations in language. At about 2–2½ years of age this echoic behaviour decreases and finally disappears (Nakanishi and Owada, 1973).

We have very little information about the very early periods of language development of the dysphasic child. But the information available suggests that at approximately 4 years of age most dysphasic children have, at least, achieved a level of expressing intentions and relations. Many of these children express these relations in a phonologically deviant form. If the results of studies of the auditory processing of these children are correct (i.e. they appear to have difficulty in differentiating and categoris-ing criterial segmental aspects of the speech sound signal) this would cause difficulty at the very early stages of development. If, as has been stated, these children are unable to relate the speech sound signal to speech acts and predications because of a symbolisation deficit (Morehead and More-head, 1974) this would cause difficulty during the period at which a basic lexicon is acquired and the period at which relations between objects and events are encoded and expressed. If imitative behaviour is a technique used by all children to try out their findings about categories and relations and these children have speech production difficulties, then the process of matching input to output will be distorted and again cause difficulties at the early stages of development. If they are unable to process more than the basic relations in sentences, because they cannot retain the information for a deeper analysis (Menyuk and Looney, 1972a) they will have difficulty during the period when the specific rules of the language used to expand noun phrases and verb phrases, mark number and tense relations within sentences, and conjoin and embed sentences are acquired.

What is being suggested is that the basis of the problem may change with time. Such a suggestion has been made previously in relation to specific developmental dyslexia (Satz *et al.*, 1971), which might be a concomitant problem of children with developmental dysphasia since the reading acquisition process presumably entails conscious awareness of linguistic categories and relations (Mattingly, 1972). Although basic auditory processing may be difficult for children with developmental dysphasia (and, indeed, may remain so for meaningless speech stimuli), speech segmental differentiation and categorisation need not continue to be the primary problem for these children in comprehension of *language*. A shift occurs in the basis upon which decisions about the meaning of utterances are made for the dysphasic and also for the normal children. That is, the basis shifts from segmental and supra-segmental (as well as gestural and contextual) to semantic and syntactic. This is clearly indicated by the ability of the children with developmental dysphasia to preserve the meaning-bearing elements, and the order in which they occur, in sentence comprehension and repetition tasks. Their knowledge of semantic and syntactic rules, however, is quite limited in comparison with normal children of the same age. The bases for these limitations may vary from child to child, and may lie in their developmental history, as well as in differences in their processing abilities.

It has been suggested that the semantic limitations of children with developmental dysphasia are related to what might be termed sub-categorisation rules; that is, knowledge of the constraints on the co-occurrence of items in a sentence (Tyack, 1969). This, in turn, requires knowledge of the differing *properties* of nouns, verbs, determiners, prepositions and adverbs. This difficulty may not only be reflected in the production of non-grammatical utterances (for example use of non-transitive verbs transitively) but may also, and to a greater extent, restrict the *range* of structures that are acquired (Morehead and Ingram, 1973). Such syntactic difficulty is reflected in these children's difficulty in encoding, storing, and retrieving syntactic regularities which go beyond the basic unmarked relations (i.e. intention, subject, verb and object). This difficulty may be due to the inability of these children to keep in mind more than the basic portions of the sentence (predicate or subject and predicate) to allow for an in-depth analysis of the sequences heard. This possibility is indicated by their more sophisticated ability to generate utterances spontaneously than to recall utterances immediately. It is possible that this difficulty results from the inability of the dysphasic children to categorise linguistic relations within the normal processing time. That is, these children may use a strategy described by Bruner (1957) as a 'constant close look' which would prohibit them from making more than a preliminary hierarchical examination of the data present in the signal. Finally, it has been suggested that the problem is one of retrieval – that is, using the knowledge of structural relations to analyse incoming data or to programme output (Weiner, 1972).

One question remains unanswered: do all children with developmental dysphasia have *all* the developmental and processing problems described above? Despite the enormous amount of research it is patently obvious that there is more to be learnt from these children. But so far the answer to the above question appears to be 'No'. Research has indicated that different children labelled as cases of developmental dysphasia have different problems, as suggested by their performance in different experimental situations. On the surface at least, the nature of their problem affects which aspects of the language they have difficulty with (structural and/or segmental), and whether their problem is one of analysis as well as output, or simply one of output. The nature of the problem appears to affect also the rate at which language develops and the direction it takes (i.e. which aspects show comparatively greater or lesser development). Although a number of suggestions have been made concerning *the* way to solve the language problems of children with developmental dysphasia, it is clear that since their language processing difficulties vary there is no consensus of the ways in which their defect can be remedied. In every instance the particular difficulties of a child should be examined and therapy adopted with more insight into his particular needs.

Acknowledgements

Part of the research for this chapter (see pp. 151–53) was carried out by the students and faculty of the Applied Psycholinguistics Program, School of Education, Boston University, and was partially supported by B.E.H. Contract No. OEC-0-749186. A preliminary report of this project has been submitted to B.E.H.

References

Bruner, J. (1957). On perceptual readiness. *Psychol. Rev.* **64**, 123–152.

Eimas, P. (1974). Linguistic Processing of Speech by Young Infants. *In* 'Language Perspectives: Acquisition, Retardation and Intervention' (R. Schiefelbusch and L. Lloyd, eds), pp. 55–73. University Park Press, Baltimore.

Farwell, C. (1972). A Note on the Production of Fricatives in Linguistically Deviant Children. Papers and Reports on Child Language Development, Stanford University, No. 4, 93–101.

Lee, L. (1966). Developmental sentence types: A method for comparing normal and deviant syntactic development. *J. Speech Hear. Dis.* **31**, 311–330.

Lee, L. (1974). 'Developmental Sentence Analysis'. Northwestern University Press, Evanston.

Leonard, L. B. (1972). What is deviant language? *J. Speech Hear. Dis.* **37**, 427–446.

Levy, C. B. and Menyuk, P. (1975). 'Cognitive and Linguistic Skills of Children with Normal and Deviant Language Development'. Paper presented at meeting of American Speech and Hearing Association, Washington, D.C.

Limber, J. (1973). The Genesis of Complex Sentences. *In* 'Cognitive Development and the Acquisition of Language' (T. Moore, ed.), pp. 169–186. Academic Press, New York.

Longhurst, T. and Schrandt, T. (1973). Linguistic analysis of children's speech: A comparison of four procedures. *J. Speech Hear. Dis.* **38**, 240–249.

Mattingly, I. G. (1972). Reading: The Linguistic Process and Linguistic Awareness. *In* 'Language by Ear and by Eye' (J. Kavanaugh and I. Mattingly, eds), pp. 133–147. M.I.T. Press, Cambridge, Mass.

Menyuk, P. (1964). Comparison of grammar of children with functionally deviant and normal speech. *J. Speech Hear. Res.* **7**, 109–121.

Menyuk, P. (1968). The role of distinctive features in the child's acquisition of phonology. *J. Speech Hear. Res.* **11**, 138–146.

Menyuk, P. (1975a). Children with Language Problems: What's the Problem? *In* Twenty-Sixth Annual Georgetown Roundtable, 'Developmental Psycholinguistics: Theory and Applications', pp. 129–144. Georgetown University Press.

Menyuk, P. (1975b). The language-impaired child: Linguistic or cognitive impairment? *Ann. N.Y. Acad. Sci.* **263**, 59–69.

Menyuk, P. (1977). 'Language and Maturation: Some Contemporary Issues', Ch. 5. M.I.T. Press, Cambridge, Mass.

Menyuk, P. and Looney, P. (1972a). A problem of language disorder: Length versus structure. *J. Speech. Hear. Res.* **15**, 264–279.

Menyuk, P. and Looney, P. (1972b). Relationships among components of the grammar in language disorder. *J. Speech Hear. Res.* **15**, 395–406.

Menyuk, P. and Looney, P. 'Speech Sound Categorization of Children with and without Language Disorders', (In preparation.)

Morehead, D. and Ingram, D. (1973). The development of base syntax in normal and linguistically deviant children. *J. Speech Hear. Res.* **16**, 330–352.

Morehead, D. and Morehead, A. (1974). From Signal to Sign: A Piagetian View of Thought and Language during the first two Years. *In* 'Language Perspectives: Acquisition, Retardation and Intervention' (R. Schiefelbusch and L. Lloyd, eds), pp. 153–190. University Park Press, Baltimore.

Nakanishi, Y. and Owada, K. (1973). Echoic utterances of children between the ages of 1 and 3 years. *J. Verbal Learn. Verbal Behav.* **12**, 658–665.

Rees, N. (1973). Auditory processing factors in language disorders: The view from Procrustes' bed. *J. Speech Hear. Dis.* **38**, 304–315.

Rosenthal, W. (1972). Auditory and Linguistic Interaction in Developmental Aphasia: Evidence from two studies of auditory processing. Papers and Reports on Child Language Development, Stanford University, No. 4, 19–34.

Satz, P., Rardin, D. and Ross, J. (1971). An evaluation of a theory of specific developmental dyslexia. *Child Devel.* **42**, 2009–2021.

Stark, J., Poppen, R. and May, M. (1967). Effects of alternation of prosodic features on the sequencing performances of aphasic children. *J. Speech Hear. Res.* **10**, 849–855.

Tallal, P. (1974). 'Is Developmental Aphasia primarily a Defect of Perception, not Language?' Paper presented at the International Neuropsychological Conference, Boston, February, 1974.

Tallal, P. and Piercy, M. (1973). Developmental aphasia: Impaired rate of non-verbal processing as a function of sensory modality. *Neuropsychologia* **11**, 389–398.

Tyack, D. (1969). 'An Analysis of the Syntactic Structures of a Child with Language Problem'. Master's Thesis, University of Illinois.

Weiner, P. (1972). The perceptual level functioning of dysphasic children: A follow-up study. *J. Speech Hear. Res.* **15**, 423–438.

Wolff, P. and Wolff, E. (1972). Correlational analysis of motor and verbal activity in young children. *Child Devel.* **43**, 1407–1411.

Treatment and Prognosis

Jean M. Cooper and Pauline Griffiths

Introduction

This chapter attempts to review the role of the speech therapist and remedial teacher in the management of children with developmental dysphasia. Some of the techniques reported here, however, could also be applicable to the treatment of children who have suffered brain damage before acquiring language.

In the context of the present paper developmental dysphasia is defined as a deficit in the acquisition of language symbols, of such severity that it interferes with the child's verbal communication. These children are often of normal, or near normal hearing, and of normal, or above normal intelligence; but they nevertheless fail to develop normal language functions. In addition to the verbal deficits they frequently show perceptual disorders in one or more sensory modalities (most frequently auditory perception) and poor control of attention, memory and motor functions (see Eisenson, 1972). The expressive language disorders frequently result from the deficits of verbal comprehension, although there are some exceptions. From the point of view of treatment, disorders which are primarily of articulation (e.g. oral dyspraxia and dysarthria) should be considered as somewhat separate problems.

Early Management

As soon as the language handicap has been diagnosed three management problems need consideration: (*i*) the appropriate time to initiate treatment; (*ii*) the person who should provide the therapy; and (*iii*) the most fitting type of programme for each individual case.

(*i*) In relation to the first problem it is important to bear in mind that there are periods of optimal learning (see Davis, 1967), and that in the case of language this period is between one-and-a-half and four-and-a-half years of age (Lenneberg, 1967). For this reason, the need to provide early treatment is of basic importance; a topic that has been discussed in several recent studies. Mylebust (1971) for example, considers that the lack of treatment at an early stage might later result in a marked retardation of other language functions such as reading and writing. Morley (1972), moreover, states that the greater the delay in the onset and use of language the greater the effect on the ultimate development of verbal communication. Morley also suggests that delayed initiation of language may prevent possible neural re-organisation of verbal functions.

(*ii*) In connection with the problem of who should provide the therapy for children with language disabilities there seems to be general agreement for a multidisciplinary approach, but it is always important to remember that all therapy whether it takes the form of medical care, perceptual training, behavioural modification or environmental control, should be directed towards achieving the basic goal of helping to develop acceptable and appropriate strategies in order to establish symbolic-linguistic behaviour (Eisenson, 1972).

There is also agreement among all those concerned with the care of language impaired children that their needs cannot be adequately met through programmes of periodic therapy, and that treatment must be included in the total daily environment of the child. This means that the assistance of the parents and Infant School teachers must be enlisted in helping these children. As most of the communication skills are acquired at home, the speech therapist should help the parents to manipulate the home environment so as to facilitate maximal conditions of learning. Frequently, the parents' reaction to this problem is to provide an increased – but non-discriminative – environmental stimulation. This should not be encouraged, as it could have deleterious effects on both the child's processes of attention and his motivation.

(*iii*) Programmes of therapy in the early stages of language handicap need to be devised to meet the requirements of each individual case. The organisation of all programmes, however, must take into consideration the basic factors known to provide maximal opportunities of learning (see Kluppel, 1972), i.e. motivation, attention, appropriate stimulus environment (i.e. stimulus conditions must be appropriate to the subject's level of performance), response appropriateness (i.e. responses should be chosen from those which are known to be part of a subject's repertoire), and reinforcement.

The basic aim in early training is to make the child attend, selectively, to the sound of the human voice. The young infant is bombarded with a variety of incoming stimuli, and from these he must select those to which he will attend. It would seem that training to attend selectively to auditory stimuli ought to be the most relevant approach for the acquisition and development of language; but in our experience we have found that attention to acoustic inputs is more difficult for the aphasic child – especially in those cases with partial hearing loss. For this reason our training is directed firstly to developing attentional skills through the visual modality, then, by manipulating motivation and reinforcement, to steadily bringing the child to direct his attention to auditorily presented stimuli and, finally, to attend and respond to the human voice. These strategies are demonstrated to the parents, stressing the following basic points: first, the necessity for a full facial presentation when speaking to the young child; second, the need to increase the intensity but decrease the rate of stimulus presentation; finally, the need to devise various games which will help to motivate the child and make him attend selectively to the presentation of the human voice.

In the early stages of therapy only simple discriminations are required, but later on the training should demand finer and more subtle discriminations of the human voice.

More recently an attempt has been made to develop symbolic function as an aid to language development. Thus, Sheridan (1969) suggests language therapy for pre-syntactic children should begin by the development of representational behaviour. It is known that representational behaviour, such as symbolic play, precedes the development of linguistic behaviour and she suggests that children who lack codes of communication should be helped by training them to imitate everyday activities. Such training will facilitate the comprehension of the functional use of objects and in turn will aid the development of concept formation (Sleigh, 1972). The first stage of imitation should be made with the use of real live objects. That is to say, the children should be given opportunity to play with domestic objects and encouraged to discover their actual purpose. In the second stage the children should be trained to recognise and imitate the use of toys, including miniature objects; later on training should be directed towards the recognition of pictures together with the development of those gestures which fit the pictorial representation. It has been stressed that all these activities must take place in the child's home environment.

Early diagnosis is being achieved more and more successfully and a growing understanding of language development is now making it possible to detect abnormalities very early in life, sometimes before the age of two years. Parallel to this, there is increasing knowledge of the means by which such disorders can be remedied and the following case history together with its management can serve to illustrate the importance of early diagnosis and early therapy.

John was referred to an assessment centre by a paediatrician at the age of three years and three months because of speech and language delay.

Birth and Development History. John's pre- and peri-natal histories were normal. Mother went into spontaneous labour at forty weeks with a normal delivery apart from the second stage, which was somewhat rapid.

John remained healthy and fed well in the neo-natal period, never had any serious illnesses or accidents and had only been admitted to hospital for tonsillectomy and myringotomy in the months just prior to his referral to the centre.

His parents began to get worried when he was between eighteen months and two years of age because he did not talk and appeared not to understand speech. This was seen in comparison to their elder son who was able to understand language and talked rather early. In contrast, however, most of John's milestones such as sitting, crawling and walking had been reached earlier than his brother's. His personality differed also from that of his brother. He seemed a somewhat stolid baby, less outgoing, but he was cuddly and enjoyed affection. He disliked going into strange places. At the time of referral he was not attempting to dress or undress himself. He was feeding himself only if his mother put the food in a spoon. He was still wearing nappies.

Family History. This was not contributory: on his maternal side there was a history of an uncle and a cousin who were said to have been 'slow in talking', but the information available was not very specific.

Assessment. Physical examination showed that John was an active child, with no neuromuscular incoordination.

He had grommets in each ear; on first examination his hearing responses were slow and it appeared he had a mild conductive hearing loss. On subsequent examination, however, this condition fluctuated, but the hearing loss was found to be only mild. Vision appeared normal.

There were no abnormal neurological signs.

The psychological assessment showed that his non-verbal abilities were consistent with his chronological age.

John held his attention very fixedly to matters of his own choice, mostly a concrete task. He was quite inflexible and could not adapt or modify his actions in response to any direction or intervention. He either ignored the presence of adults or else he moved away. He could not understand the concept of reward, i.e. that he would get a sweet if he carried out a specific request; the reward, to be effective, had to be part of the task itself.

John demonstrated to some extent understanding of representational toys by classifying objects, e.g. putting all the cars in a row and all the beds in another row. There was, however, no attempt to play imaginatively with the toys or even to relate them in ways which might suggest symbolic meaning. He could not match toys and pictures. Verbal comprehension was poor. He followed familiar situational phrase patterns but was only able to select three test objects in response to naming. His expressive language consisted of the sound 'mu' which was used always when he wanted something. Apart from this and the use of varying intonation on vowel sounds, there was nothing else systematic; in effect he had no communicative vocal language.

Therapy Programme. John attended regularly with his mother. His father could only attend very occasionally. The mother appeared very cooperative and anxious to be involved in the treatment. This involved the development of a better control of attention, and symbolic understanding, as well as attempts to improve language comprehension and verbal expression.

Attention Control. This was one of John's greatest learning handicaps at first and it was necessary to help his mother to recognise his difficulty, and to gain his attention and help him to control it in order for him to benefit from a learning situation. Games were devised to encourage and attract John's facial attention, even if fleetingly at first. Over a period of several weeks attention improved in so far that he seldom disregarded the therapist, although his attention still shifted very rapidly. He was rewarded for any attempt to focus his attention, however short the duration. By the age of five John's attention had improved very considerably, and he has become a much more accessible and teachable child.

Symbolic Understanding. It was necessary to demonstrate to John's mother how to develop some imaginative play by using a large doll or Teddy bear. His mother appeared to have a good understanding of what was required and although at first much of the play with Teddy consisted of John's imitating mother's play, e.g. putting Teddy to bed, giving Teddy a drink, etc., gradually he was able to carry out some play sequences initiated by himself. After 4 or 5 months the therapist introduced the idea of playing with smaller size toy material.

Within a year John's play was much more imaginative; he could match toys to pictures and subsequently picture to picture, matching objects with increasingly dissimilar features, e.g. pictures of cup and beaker. He then became able to categorise objects by use, e.g. things we wear, things we eat, etc., thus demonstrating not only an understanding of the symbols but also a gradual movement from perceptual to conceptual understanding. By the age of five this had developed very successfully.

Verbal Comprehension. As John's attention control showed some improvement, he gradually responded to the spoken word more readily and was able to select objects by naming. The therapist then guided his mother into helping him to relate two named objects, e.g. put the *car* in the *box*, put the *cup* on the *chair*, etc.

John then progressed to being able to select objects by verbal description of their use, e.g. which is the one you wash in (basin), which is the one we ride in (car), etc; and he was able to link names and adjectives, e.g. which is the *big ball*, which is the *red shoe*, etc. At the age of five he was still having difficulty in understanding phrases which carried three or more concepts, but during the following year this improved so that he could cope with verbal directions containing up to 4 'operative' words, including abstractions such as size, length, passive tenses and negatives.

Expressive Language. This aspect of communication was not emphasised in the therapy situation at first, and it was necessary for the mother to accept that the other aspects such as attention control and the building up of symbolic understanding had to precede this area of development. During the first year of therapy John began to use a great deal of jargon and gradually some true verbal labels emerged; his mother was encouraged to reinforce the jargon utterances by feeding back the appropriate word or phrase. As true language developed it became evident that John was having a great deal of difficulty in phonetic organisation and sequencing; this unfortunately interfered with social communication as the listener was often dependent upon contextual clues in order to understand.

Summary. John made good progress in all aspects of language. At the age of six he was well up to his chronological level in many areas of intellectual ability but still showing some difficulty with abstract thought processes. The most suitable educational placement was thought to be a small class in a normal school, where he could get a great deal of individual help for his language difficulty. Fortunately John was referred for help at a reasonably early age (though a year earlier might have prevented difficulties in school placement). In view of the fact that therapy, with the help of the parents, began at an early age it was possible to emphasise the areas directly involved in the learning of linguistic concepts, so that these could be developed in relation to the child's meaningful experience.

Some Educational Considerations

When dysphasic children are ready for formal education, speech therapy and teaching may be effectively merged in the overall planning of remediation. Traditional concepts of teaching, therapy, intelligence, education and even language should not be allowed to jeopardise an objective and radical approach to the problem. In common with many other aspects of education, most methods of remediation have been developed pragmatically. Teachers and therapists have to deal with the reality presented by learning problems which often have not been studied in depth or where the condition has not been generally acknowledged.

DESCRIPTION OF LEARNING PROBLEMS PRESENTED

Characteristically, these children show a wide range of levels of functioning, and also of learning disability, both within and between individuals.

Reading, writing and number learning is usually severely affected. Some children may learn limited 'drills' relatively easily but comprehension has to be developed slowly and laboriously. Memory limitations are common, particularly in relation to the ordering and sequencing of material. In a very few children storage of symbolic material is so limited that learning is made virtually impossible.

This may be illustrated by the two following cases:

Pamela

C.A. 6 years 1 month; M.A. 5 years 6 months

	Equivalent age level
Motor skills	6 yrs
Social development	3 yrs
Auditory discrimination	Untestable
Auditory memory	2 yrs 7 mths
Receptive vocabulary	Under 1 yr 6 mths
Verbal comprehension	1 yr
Expressive vocabulary	2 yrs 2 mths
Expressive language	1 yr
Articulation	Untestable
Visual motor skills	5 yrs 6 mths
Visual memory	5 yrs 8 mths
School attainments	Nil

Wayne

C.A. 6 years 11 months; M.A. 6 years

	Equivalent age level
Motor skills	5 yrs 8 mths
Social development	3 yrs 2 mths
Auditory discrimination	Under 4 yrs
Auditory memory	Under 4 yrs
Receptive vocabulary	2 yrs 1 mth
Verbal comprehension	3 yrs 1 mth
Expressive vocabulary	Untestable
Expressive language	2 yrs 4 mths
Articulation	Under 3 yrs 1 mth
Visual motor skills	4 yrs 6 mths
School attainments	Nil

In addition to the various perceptual difficulties described in other chapters in this book there may be problems of attention, concentration, tendency to perseveration and restless behaviour. Although most commonly children are friendly, affectionate and cheerfully heedless, some may show wilful determination, reckless fearlessness, aggressive outbursts, obsessional behaviour and occasionally emotional detachment.

Amongst this variety of features only one characteristic seems to appear consistently: a difficulty with temporal ordering which is readily shown by an inability to reproduce a rhythmic beat. The children may be able to follow a steady, moderately slow beat, but anything more complicated is virtually impossible without a prolonged training. Difficulties are also encountered with singing in tune, and most children can only begin to do this at the age of eight or nine after careful teaching (Griffiths, 1972).

From the educational point of view it is more important to identify the types of disability shown by individual children than to reach a formal diagnosis of developmental dysphasia. Once the difficulties have been outlined it is profitable to group together those handicaps which are amenable to the same teaching approach. Special schools vary both in the facilities they can offer and in the range of handicap within a given category which they are prepared to accept. It is important to distinguish between a clinical and an educational diagnosis. The latter will invariably be broader but confusion can arise when a child fails to respond to a particular method of remedial teaching. The assumption that the diagnostic category bears a direct relation to the teaching method sometimes leads, in the case of failure, to a claim of mis-diagnosis. This can result in months and even years of delay in placing the child in an appropriate school. It is often more important to change the teaching method than to change the diagnosis.

Among a sample of several hundred 6-year-old children, described as dysphasic or with specific language disorder and referred for special educational treatment, the following five groups could be distinguished. None of these children had a major mental or physical handicap.

1 Children who demonstrate normal hearing on audiometry but who show little or no ability to comprehend or use speech. They are bright and alert, and show a keen awareness of their environment; they relate cause and effect and demonstrate appropriate (if immature) social behaviour. They may be socially dependent but are usually well adjusted and keen to communicate and may show considerable ingenuity in developing ways of doing this. Some acquire skill in drawing and seem to find this a satisfying form of self-expression. There is a moderate use of mime and communicative gesture, and their ability to form concepts, enter into imaginative situations and empathise with others is present although slow to develop. There is usually no evidence of motor impairment although the characteristic difficulty with rhythmic tasks is apparent. In general, there are more girls than boys in this group.

2 Children with hearing loss which varies from mild to profound and who, despite sound amplification and the normal methods of teaching the deaf, have failed to acquire comprehension or use of spoken language. There may be a history of maternal rubella (with other associated handicaps), long and difficult birth, prematurity or very low birth weight (4 lb or less). Motor coordination is usually good but some have a history of mild spasticity noted soon after birth. Visual handicaps such as a squint may also be present. These children often use a great deal of communicative gesture and mime, but behaviour may be marked by hyperactivity and gross immaturity.

3 In this group are children whose verbal comprehension is normal or just below their mental age, but whose expressive language may be absent or else severely retarded. Their vocabulary may be limited to about one hundred words which are used singly. If there is an attempt to join words their speech is usually telegraphic. Verbs may be used only in the present tense with omission of inflectional endings and most auxiliaries. Prepositions may be missing and use of pronouns confused.

Interrogative and negative forms may still be immature and speech consist mainly of short, simple active declaratives with frequent use of 'and'. A phonological disorder is usually present and speech may be unintelligible to all but their immediate family. Nevertheless, communication is usually attempted through a patient persistence with 'speech' even when this consists of no more than grunts.

A few of these children have a gross articulatory impairment accompanied by dribbling and difficulties with chewing and swallowing. Most show evidence of a general though mild motor impairment and are clumsy and awkward. At the age of 8 or 9 they may still have difficulties in learning to ride a bicycle, jump with both feet off the ground, catch a large ball or climb stairs with a foot on successive steps. In spite of this, they are generally very active and appear to enjoy boisterous, unorganised activity into which they hurl themselves – often with a surprising degree of success. In this group there are usually more boys than girls.

4 This group is very similar to the last, but in spite of a late onset (3–4 years) spoken language develops relatively rapidly and by the age of 7–8 years there may be only residual traces of difficulty. These children, however, show severe difficulties in learning to read. In spite of highly skilled individual teaching, progress is extremely slow and shows all the characteristic features of developmental dyslexia. Problems of fine motor coordination may be relatively severe but general cognitive function is good and intelligence levels often well above average.

5 The children in this group may develop a grasp of the mechanics of speech but, in spite of adequate phonology and grammar, their use of speech is often imitative, stereotyped and irrelevant. They may demonstrate a level of performance on certain intelligence tests which is appropriate for their age, and a mechanical ability to read and write. Their learning skills, however, in terms of comprehension, ability to form concepts, abstractions and generalisations, are even more severely affected than in non-verbal children. They may be very observant of the physical dimensions of objects, e.g. colour, outline shape, movement, etc., and they may show good rote learning ability and have good motor coordination. These children are frequently obsessional and seem to show a preference for maps, charts, diagrams, clocks, dials and figures. They relate better to adults than to children of the same age, to whom they are mostly indifferent. They do not indulge in imaginative play but occupy themselves alone with their current obsession. In the classroom they are quietly eccentric but not usually disruptive.

This descriptive grouping of children must, of course, be seen only as a very broad categorisation of the problems, which are presented in the classroom. The diversity of disorder is great and gradations occur within and between the groups.

EDUCATIONAL IMPLICATIONS

The development of remedial methods for dysphasic children rests on two basic considerations:

1 The needs of the child as an individual and as a member of society.

2 The demands of society as communicated through education. The needs of the child will include:

Communicative contact

Validation and identity

Time and opportunity to develop his abilities
   to the full.

Cultural demands include:

Communication through speech

Social acceptability

Competence in basic skills of self-care
   and development of reading, writing and numerical abilities.

Communication with others, and mediation in thought processes, are the main functions of language which may be roughly defined as a systematic verbal code. It is well known that some form of inner representation is a necessary part of cognitive function. This does not have to be verbal but, as Furth (1966) has shown, much of the development of intelligence, including the ability to conceptualise, relate and generalise, depends on the degree of development of this codifying system. It is not known precisely what form this code may take in different individuals and the common designation of 'inner language' may be misleading if this is taken to imply an inner *verbal* capacity. For this reason a less specific 'codifying system' seems preferable.

Speech is the arbitrarily imposed function of a particular cultural environment. It is normally a manifestation of the inner codifying system and is used to express it. In children with specific language disability, however, a separation between these two systems can occur. This distinction is fundamental to remedial teaching and is frequently an area of considerable confusion and conflict for educators.

Communication is a central part of education, and the manner of teaching is mostly verbal. Furthermore, the educational aim of enabling children to function as normally as possible within society must include normal verbal communication. The highly formal lexical, syntactical and phonological conventions of a given language will not be learnt naturally by a dysphasic child nor by any teaching that involves natural acquisition methods. But this does not mean that he is incapable of learning them.

Efforts to achieve this have in some cases led to extreme emphasis on speech for its own sake. For example 'labels' may be taught in an attempt to build up a vocabulary, but in doing so one could fail to consider the importance of linguistic structure which is much more relevant to intellectual growth. Children may be taught to recite strings of words which are entirely dependent upon specific situations and can never be generalised or used spontaneously. Even more detrimental are the attempts made to prevent children from using their own natural means of expression and communication. Some teachers wish to stop completely the use of gesture, which is a natural concomitant of normal speech, and they may reject the child's attempts at verbalisation if it is not expressed in grammatical form. Such efforts to produce 'speech' at the expense of spontaneous communication may deprive the child of the opportunity to develop his powers of symbolic thought. Remediation should rather be concerned with fostering the child's particular mode of thought, helping him to verbalise as far as possible, and teaching linguistic conventions through which he can express himself in a socially acceptable manner.

A language handicap is also a social handicap (Rutter and Martin, 1972). Poor verbal comprehension may insulate the child from the subtleties of social interaction and his own frustration at his inability to express himself can lead to a cumulative situation of social immaturity, misunderstanding and exasperation. Because representational play is usually slow to develop there is a late onset of role play and the development of what Werner (Langer, 1970) has referred to as 'perspectivism'. This is the ability to see another's point of view and to link the development of symbolic thinking to self-awareness and awareness of others. An example of this is the difficulty many dysphasic children have in understanding family relationships. Eight- or nine-year-old children may readily and adequately use the terms 'brothers' and 'sisters' but they are quite unable to see themselves in that role. Similarly, they may find it impossible to grasp that 'mummy' can also fulfil the roles of daughter and sister even when they have no difficulty in understanding these terms in relation to themselves. An understanding of interpersonal roles and a self-awareness in relation to others, as well as the ability to sympathise and empathise, are all contributory to social behaviour which the child may need help to develop.

The educational task may perhaps be summarised as follows: the child needs time to develop, and the ten or eleven years of statutory schooling could be extended at both ends in order to provide greater benefits to him. The development of intellectual functioning is more important than imposed 'speech', but in its turn it depends to some extent on the acquisition of a communication code. As Lewis (1965) has stated, 'Cognitive immaturity has long been thought, and rightly, to be a cause of linguistic retardation. It is no less important to recognise that linguistic immaturity may be a cause of cognitive retardation'. The communication code to be taught must be that of society but the child will not learn it by natural means, i.e. as a result of normal environmental experience.

Because of the uneven levels of functioning of dysphasic children, educational approaches may be made through the more highly developed areas. The approach needs to be

(a) Multi-sensory – avoiding reliance on the auditory modality.

(b) Within the limits of the child's level of symbolic development.

(c) Simplified and structured. New material has to be presented in the smallest possible steps and the relationship to what has already been learnt pointed out. At first the teacher must be responsible for the ordering of information so that a logical sequence may be developed – e.g. even the simplest categorisation of objects is not possible until the concept of 'same' and 'different' has been taught.

(*d*) Often a reversal of normal teaching procedures may be necessary, e.g. the child may be helped to speak by first learning to read; the 'enriched' environment normally considered to be linguistically stimulating may have to be drastically restricted and controlled in order to make it meaningful to the child.

EDUCATIONAL APPROACHES

Many writers have stressed the importance of a multi-sensory approach (McGinnis, 1963; Monsees, 1972; Hutt, 1973). Intelligent children with normal hearing who fail to learn language by aural/oral means will learn if a visual and kinaesthetic approach is used. Visual material can also be made relatively static so that it not only presents the temporal patterning of speech (which may be a special difficulty for dysphasic children) in a spatial dimension, but also gives the child time to understand it. Written language, however, loses the dynamic aspect of speech and it is very difficult to demonstrate the temporality of verb tenses even with the aid of pictures.

Verbal language can be presented visually by three means:

1 Sign language
2 Lip (or speech) reading
3 Reading and writing.

With the aid of sign language speech can be presented visually and dynamically. If a sign system – capable of representing morphological processes – such as the Paget Gorman Sign System (Crystal and Craig, 1978) is used, it can be consistently related to speech and writing and therefore can be applied as a method of teaching different aspects of language. This system is also mentioned by Conn (1974) in his discussion of the possibilities of reducing the arbitrariness of language forms. This is an important consideration for children who, even after starting school, may need a simplification of the symbolic aspect of language.

Stages in the development of symbolic function as manifested by representational play have been suggested by Sheridan (1972), Sleigh (1972) and Lowe (1975). Language development in its spoken and written forms involves increasing complexity of symbolic association (Hutt, 1973). At the beginning, a radical simplification of language in every aspect – symbolic, semantic, syntactic and phonemic – may be necessary. Material may have to be three-dimensional (real objects, miniatures, Action Men, etc.), and it is important not to over-stimulate or confuse the child with too much at once.

Attempts to simplify language have led some workers, e.g. McGinnis (1963) and Monsees (1972), to approach the problem first through the phonological level (this being relatively demonstrable and therefore 'easiest') and then work through the morphology to syntax. The dysphasic child finds extreme difficulty in acquiring speech but by contrast he has a relatively well-developed codifying system. For these reasons some authors have found that it is easier to teach morphology and syntax through writing (e.g. Lea, 1970; Conn, 1971; Thomas, 1972). Lea and Conn relate word classes to colours so that in the early stages children can learn the grammatical features through a colour pattern. A minimum vocabulary is chosen in order to limit the number of words and concepts which the child is required to learn. It should represent the basic essentials of what is needed in and out of the classroom, and would provide a measure of consistency amongst those who speak to the child.

The language failure is not due to a linguistically deprived environment; therefore it is not amenable to environmental enrichment and stimulation as the sole means of treatment. In fact children who are subjected to stimulation and demands that are beyond their perceptual powers may react with disorganised, disturbed or withdrawn behaviour. In some cases this may be an attempt to avoid failure but in others it seems to be a generalised reaction to excitation and distress.

Linguistic concepts, on the other hand, can only be taught in relation to the child's meaningful experience. In order to do this the teacher has to control the environment and the child's degree of involvement. In extreme cases of distractibility, it has been suggested that the child may need periods in a small enclosed area with bare walls. At first, he is not expected to distinguish what is relevant from a background of 'noise' – he is given no option in what he attends to. This is also one of the functions of a highly structured teaching programme – in addition it serves as an attention-training scheme.

Programmes designed to accelerate general development in terms of 'learning readiness' and the training of sub-skills have proved disappointing in the subsequent learning of linguistic skills. There seems to be no evidence that transfer occurs and attention control, fine motor coordination, spatial and auditory discrimination can be more successfully developed in the process of direct language intervention.

Because of the diversity of learning problems that occur it is unlikely that any given group will display uniform difficulties. In spite of this there are advantages to be obtained from group teaching. It offers a more natural situation for the child, and provides opportunities for social learning. Group teaching removes the pressure of a continually one-to-one situation and offers the teacher/therapist greater scope for general manipulation of the environment. It is essential, however, that teaching be prescriptive, and the child's changing needs and priorities must be continually assessed, and when necessary he should be provided with additional individual work.

This approach to remediation is designed to achieve aural/oral communication wherever possible. To some it may sound like 'anti-education'. It is indeed the antithesis of heuristic, child-centred education. In contrast with pre-school remediation it is frequently *not* developmental because of the huge variation in the functional levels that develops as the child gets older. It is contrived, rigid and deliberately limiting. It does, however, succeed where ordinary educational methods have failed, and if special education is to be something more than a euphemism the comparison is irrelevant.

Nevertheless, it must not be forgotten that these methods are only a starting point. They can be used as long as necessary, modified, used selectively or even abandoned. Education consists of a great deal more than language remediation but little more is available to the child who has not first been taught how to learn.

Outcome and Prognosis

Very few studies on prognosis are available and indeed many more are needed.

The present writer reviewed 49 children who had been pupils at the John Horniman School (Griffiths, 1969). This is a special school which offers educational treatment for children with severe language disabilities from 5 to 9 years of age. These children received, on average, nearly two years' special education and on leaving approximately one-third were able to return to ordinary schools, a third went to other special schools such as Delicate, E.S.N., etc. (often depending on local availability) and a third required continued education as severely language-handicapped.

Follow-up studies showed that although in many cases spoken language appeared 'normal' the children were failing educationally. A surprising number of class teachers said they did not even know the child had ever been considered handicapped or received special education in spite of the reports available. Some had made little progress in reading since the end of their special education; and some of the children who attended ordinary schools (the least linguistically handicapped) showed behaviour disorder and other symptoms of stress which had not been apparent before.

The children in ordinary schools had shown no sustained progress despite the fact that their attainments on leaving the special school were only a year behind their mental age. Although their linguistic difficulties had been apparently resolved, they nevertheless possessed a persistent and hidden disability which continued to require special educational treatment.

The presence of persistent disability in children with delayed speech development has been confirmed by Garvie and Gordon (1973). They reviewed 58 children of whom 25 were attending ordinary schools. Of the 13 whose language was within normal limits, 6 had reading and writing difficulties and a relationship between this and behavioural disturbance was noted.

In a follow-up study of 10 young adults undertaken by Moor House School (1969), it was found that in spite of severe linguistic handicap (reading age at about an 8- to 9-year-old level and spoken language attainments usually well below this), nearly all were successfully employed. Although they were generally well accepted by their work-mates, many were lonely and the development of social contacts constituted their greatest problem.

In terms of the five groups previously described, those in groups three and four (mainly with expressive language difficulties) are the most likely to be able to return to an ordinary school, although the persistent reading and writing difficulties of group four will generally require special help.

Children in groups one and two (with comprehension and expressive disabilities) can attain a relatively good standard of reading and writing and usually acquire enough speech for simple communication. Development of spoken language is greatly helped by using the Paget Gorman Sign System (*loc. cit.*) as it aids recall of morphological and syntactical features. But because of their severe difficulties in speech comprehension these children are never likely to attend ordinary classes; those in group two, however, may do well in oral schools for the deaf.

Group five, some of whom may use speech in an automatic manner but who show little or no evidence of conceptual thought, present severe educational difficulties. Although they may be able to learn the mechanics of speech relatively easily, comprehension of underlying processes fails to develop and they are unable to generalise or utilise previous experience. All new material has to be learnt afresh and what has been acquired before may interfere with, rather than assist, the process. Their thinking is rigid and they may replace one obsessive interest with another. Although verbally more proficient, these children may not achieve the intellectual or socially acceptable levels of other groups.

References

Berry, M. F. and Eisenson, J. (1956). 'Speech Disorders'. Appleton-Century-Crofts, New York.

Berry, M. F. (1969). 'Language Disorders of Children'. Appleton-Century-Crofts, New York.

Conn, P. J. (1971). 'Remedial Syntax (John Horniman School Working Papers on Language Therapy No. 1)'. Invalid Children's Aid Association, London.

Conn, P. J. (1974). The interrelations of alternatives in symbolic representation. *Br. J. Dis. Commun.* **9**, 92.

Cooper, J., Moodley, M. and Reynell, J. (1974). Intervention programmes for pre-school children with delayed language development. *Br. J. Dis. Commun.* **9**, 81–91.

Crystal, D. and Craig, E. (1978). Contrived Sign Language. *In* 'Sign Language of the Deaf: psychological, linguistic and sociological perspectives' (I. M. Schlesinger and L. Namir, eds). Academic Press, London and New York.

Davis, D. R. (1967). Family processes in mental retardation. *Amer. J. Psychiat.* **124**, 340–350.

Eisenson, J. (1966). Perceptual disturbances in children with central nervous system dysfunction. Implications for language development. *Br. J. Dis. Commun.* **1**, 21–32.

Eisenson, J. (1972). 'Aphasia in Children'. Harper and Row, New York.

Furth, H. G. (1966). 'Thinking without Language'. Free Press, New York.

Garvie, M. and Gordon, N. (1973). A follow-up study of children with disorders of speech development. *Br. J. Dis. Commun.* **8**, 17.

Griffiths, C. P. S. (1969). A follow-up study of children with disorders of speech. *Br. J. Dis. Commun.* **4**, 46.

Griffiths, P. (1972). 'Developmental Aphasia: an Introduction'. Invalid Children's Aid Association, London.

Hutt, E. (1973). 'Systematic Sequential Instruction (John Horniman School Working Papers on Language Therapy No. 2)'. Invalid Children's Aid Association, London.

Kluppel, D. D. (1972). *In* 'Educational Management of Speaking and Listening. Principles of Childhood Language Disabilities' (J. V. Irwin and M. Marge, eds), pp. 315–327. Appleton-Century-Crofts, New York.

Langer, J. (1970). Werner's Comparative Organismic Theory. *In* 'Carmichael's Manual of Child Psychology' Vol. 1. (P. H. Mussen, ed). Wiley, New York.

Lea, J. (1970), 'The Colour Pattern Scheme: A Method of Remedial Language Teaching', Moor House School, Oxted, England.

Lenneberg, E. (1967). 'Biological Foundations of Language'. John Wiley and Sons, New York.

Lewis, M. M. (1965). 'Impairment of Language in Relation to General Development in Children with Communication Problems'. Pitman Medical Publications Co., London.

Lowe, M. (1975). Trends in the development of representational play in infants from one to three years—an observational study. *J. Child Psychol. Psychiat.* **16**, 33.

McGinnis, M. (1963). 'Aphasic Children'. Alex. Graham Bell Association for the Deaf, Inc., Washington, D.C.

Monsees, E. K. (1972). 'Structured Language for Children with Special Language Learning Problems'. Children's Hearing and Speech Centre, Children's Hospital of the District of Columbia, Washington, D.C.

Moor House School (1969). Follow-up Report. Oxted, Surrey, England.

Morley, M. E. (1972). 'The Development and Disorders of Speech in Childhood'. Churchill Livingston, Edinburgh and London.

Mykelbust, H. R. (1971). *In* 'Childhood Aphasia: Identification, Diagnosis, Remediation. Handbook of Speech Pathology and Audiology' (L. E. Travis, ed). Appleton-Century-Crofts, New York.

Rutter, M. and Martin, J. A. M. (1972). 'The Child with Delayed Speech'. Clinics in Developmental Medicine, No. 43, S.I.M.P. Heinemann Medical, London.

Sheridan, M. D. (1969). Playthings in the development of language. *Health Trends* **1**, 7–10.

Sheridan, M. D. (1972). The Child's Acquisition of Codes for Personal and Inter-personal Communication. *In* 'The Child with Delayed Speech', Clinics in Developmental Medicine, No. 43 (M. Rutter and J. A. M. Martin, eds), S.I.M.P. Heinemann Medical, London.

Sleigh, G. (1972). A study of some symbolic processes in young children. *Br. J. Dis. Commun.* **7**, 163–175.

Thomas, F. J. (1972). 'Guidelines'. Woodford Educational Publications, 178 Snakes Lane, Woodford Green, Essex, England.

SUBJECT INDEX